Evaluation and Treatment of Pediatric Feeding Disorders: from NICU to Childhood

Cheri Fraker, CCC/SLP,CLC
Laura Walbert, CCC/SLP,CLC

Foreword by Mark Fishbein, MD

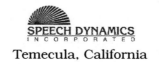

Temecula, California

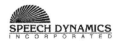

Published by
Speech Dynamics, Inc.
1-800-337-9049

Copyright ©2003 by Cheri Fraker and Laura Walbert

ISBN #
Manufactured in the United States of America
First Edition

All rights reserved. No part of this book may be reproduced
or transmitted in any form or by any means, electronic or mechanical, including
photocopying, recording or by any information storage and retrieval system without
written permission from the author.

For information regarding other publications, videos, audios,
CD's or therapeutic tools, visit www.speechdynamics.com
or call 1-800-337-9049.

Table of Contents

A Note to the Reader
Acknowledgements
Foreword by Mark Fishbein, MD
How to Use This Book
Introduction
Why Feeding Therapy? Ask the Doctor

Chapter One, Swallowing 1
What's Up, Doc?. 1
Therapist to Therapist 2
Ask Yourself These Questions 2
Suggestions for Therapy. 5
Emily: Aspiration Case Study 6
The Swallowing Sequence 8
Swallowing and the Nervous System 9
Suck-Swallow-Breathe Sequence 11
Phases of Deglutition 12

Chapter Two, Aspiration. 15
Aspiration in Infants and Children 15
Aspiration and the Lungs 17
Signs and Symptoms of Aspiration. 18
Assessment of Aspiration 18
Treatment of Aspiration. 21
Aspiration and Tracheotomy Tubes 25

Chapter Three, The Premature Infant:
Evaluation and Treatment:. 27
Practical Guidelines for Working with the Premature Infant 27
Case Study: Jeremy, a NICU Infant 29
Evaluation and Treatment 32
Assessing State Level 32
Assessing Oral Reflexes 34
Assessing Nutritive Sucking/Swallowing 35
Assessing Infant Cues 36
Facilitating a Calm State and Stability 36
When is Baby Ready for Nippling? 38

Chapter Four, The Premature Infant:
Medical Reference Guide: 41

Prematurity and the Risk Factors 41
Antenatal Steroid Therapies for the Mother 42
Complications of Pregnancy and Delivery 43
    Abruptio Placentae 43
    Antepartum Conditions 44
    Apnea of Prematurity 45
    Bronchopulmonary Dysplasia 45
    Congenital Diaphragmatic Hernia 46
    Disseminated Intravascular Coagulation (DIC) . . . 47
    HELLP Syndrome 48
    Hematocrit Level 48
    Hyperbilirubinemia 49
    Intracerebellar Hemorrhage 49
    Intracranial Hemorrhage 50
    Meconium Aspiration Syndrome (MAS) 50
    Meningitis 51
    Necrotizing Enterocolitis (NEC) 51
    Periventricular and Intraventricular Hemorrhage (IVH) . 52
    Periventricular Leukomalacia 53
    Persistent Pulmonary Hypertension of the Newborn (PPHN) . 54
    Placenta Previa 54
    Pneumonia 55
    Polycythemia 56
    Polyhydraminos 56
    Premature Rupture of the Membranes (PROM) . . . 56
    Respiratory Distress Syndrome (RDS), or Hyaline Membrane Disease . 56
    Retinopathy of Prematurity 57
    Sepsis 58
    Subarchnoid Hemorrhage 58
    Thrombocytopenia 58
    Umbilical Cord Prolapse 58
Medications 59

Chapter Five, Evaluation and Treatment of the Newborn:
Typical Oral-Motor Development of the Term Infant 62

Oral Reflexes 62
Feeding Skills by Age and Volume Per Feeding 65
A Word about Juice 71
Bottle Feeding Guidelines 72
Infant Formula Guide 72
Introduction of Semi-Solids and Solid Foods 74
Spoon Feeding Guidelines 75
Cup Drinking 75
Infant Appetite 76

Chapter Six, Breastfeeding. 77

Therapist Chat 77
Case Example: Grace 77
Nipple Confusion: Fact or Fiction? 81
Breastmilk. 82
The Mechanics of Breastfeeding 83
Advantages of Breastfeeding 83
Advantages to the Mother. 83
Breastfeeding Trends 83
Complications 84
Breastfeeding the Special Needs Infant 84
Recommendations for the Mother of a Premature Infant 85
Kangaroo Care 86
Pacifiers 86

Chapter Seven, Treatment Programs 87

Chat Time: Specific Infant Treatment Strategies. 87
Nipple Choice 88
Endurance Problems 88
Poor Suck. 89
Poor Coordination of the Suck-Swallow-Breathe Sequence . . . 90
Oral-Facial Hypersensitivity/Early Feeding Aversion. 91
Oral-Motor Therapy is More than the Nuk Brush 92
Drooling Management 94

Chapter Eight, Evaluation and Treatment of Feeding Aversion. 95

Red Flags for Future Feeding Difficulties or Feeding Aversion . . . 95
Treatment Guidelines, "The Rules". 96
What Type of Aversion? Mild vs. Extreme Selectivity, Typical Features . 99
Setting the Tone: Environmental Intervention for Feeding Disorders . . 100
Strategies to Increase Texture in Foods 101
The Right Food at the Right Time: Food Chaining 102
Tips for Successful Food Chaining 106
What if the Child Refuses a Food in the Chain? 107
For Parents: What is Food Chaining? 110
Sample Food Chains 111
Food Chain Calendar 114

Chapter Nine, Special Topics. 116

Chat Time 116
Cleft Lip and Palate. 116
Tracheomalacia and Laryngomalacia 117
Down Syndrome. 118
Cardiac Conditions 119
Hypoxic Ischemic Encephalopathy (HIE). 121
Shaken Baby Syndrome and Brain Injury 123
Seizure Disorder 125
Cerebral Palsy 125
Esophageal Atresia and Tracheoesophageal Fistula 128

Autistic Spectrum Disorder 128
Cancer 130

Chapter Ten, Nutrition and Digestive Disorders **131**
The Digestive Tract 131
Non-Oral Feedings 132
Surgical Management of Reflux: Is a Nissen Fundolication Needed?. . 134
Transition to Oral Feedings 134
Parenteral Nutrition 135
Disorders and Dysphagia: Reference Guide. 135
Failure to Thrive 136
Treatment of FTT 137
Gastroesophageal Reflux/Chalasia 139
Eosinophilic Gastroenteritis. 142
Cyclic Vomiting Syndrome 142
Pyloric Stenosis 144
Duodenal Atresia and Stenosis 144
Midgut Volvus 144
Hirschsprung's Disease 145
Malabsorption 145
Celiac Disease 146
Lactose Intolerance. 146
Ulcerative Colitis 147
Crohn's Disease 148
Dumping Syndrome 148

Chapter Eleven, Additional Resources **149**
Comparison of Disposable and Market Brand Nipples 149
General Feeder Instructions Prior to Starting
a Behavioral Feeding Program. 156
Evaluation of Feeding Skills: Infant/Child. 159
Fraker-Walbert Feeding History/Referral Guide 162
Inpatient Oral-Motor/Feeding Evaluation: Premature Infant . . . 167
Feeding Team Clinic Evaluation and Recommendations Summary . . 170
Inpatient Daily Team Meeting Form 171
Inpatient Daily Feeding Evaluation Form 172

References

A Note to the Reader

This book contains only suggestions for evaluation and treatment of pediatric feeding disorders. Please note that no book can take the place of complete and thorough assessment and treatment program by an experienced speech pathologist/pediatric oral feeding specialist with the support of a pediatric feeding team. The therapist should share all significant findings/concerns with the child's pediatrician or primary care physician, consult occupational or physical therapy for assistance with positioning for safe oral intake and a dietitian for recommendations regarding nutrition.

Acknowledgements

Thank you, thank you.... Our thanks to Dr. Mark Fishbein, pediatric gastroenterologist and Dr. Jeri Beth Karkos, pediatric rehab medicine, from the SIU School of Medicine, Hilary Morelock, CCC/SLP and Jennifer Chalekson, RD for their contributions to this project. Thank you to our families, our colleagues in speech, occupational and physical therapy and the nursing staff at St. John's Children's Hospital in Springfield, Illinois for their support and for all they have taught us over the years of working together.

Thank you to Valerie Jones, RN, Cheryl Wilson, RN and Brenda Yale, RN for taking the time to teach us about feeding and caring for premature babies. Their information and guidance have been invaluable to our department.

Cheri would like to thank Elliot Batten for making me laugh and for helping me develop food chaining. A special thanks to our friend Frank Goldacker, Ph.D, from Eastern Illinois University. Frank, you started it all!

Please feel free to contact us at **preemietalk@insightbb.com.**

Foreword

Eating is something most people take for granted. Babies are born and instinctively know how to suck enabling them to meet their nutritional needs. Children progress through the different stages, mastering each one as they go along from bottle or breastfeeding all the way up to solid foods.

Feeding is not only a natural part of life, but also a vital part of life. Without the ability to meet our nutritional needs in some way, our life is in jeopardy. One cannot exist without nutrition. That is why a feeding problem changes the way a person views eating. It is no longer something that is given little thought. The feeding problem is now all encompassing. Well meaning family and friends give well intentioned advice which may make the family feel worse when it doesn't work for them. This is a lonely place to be.

By the time a family seeks medical attention they may be exhausted, angry, and even desperate. They may be defensive and feel guilty about the situation. A child presenting to the medical community will have both physical and emotional needs. Medical personnel will be treating not just the child but also the entire family. All members of the family are affected by a feeding problem. Family life now revolves around mealtimes. Something a family once took for granted is now the main focus of family life.

Feeding problems can develop at any time in a child's life. Premature infants have various feeding problems depending on their gestational age at birth. Children of all ages can have feeding issues as a result of a medical condition or behavior issue.

As a pediatric gastroenterologist, I have been asked to care for many infants and children with feeding disorders. These cases are often complex and challenging. It is rewarding to see a child transition mealtime from a stressful battle or struggle to a pleasurable event.

At this institution, our feeding team has been able to accomplish this task on a routine basis. Our feeding team has thrived due in large part to the will power and commitment of the speech-language pathologists. Their "expanded" roles on the feeding team include assessment of oral motor skills, oral sensory issues, deglutition (swallow) and behaviors surrounding the feeding process. These individuals devise the meal and snack time protocol including schedule, food type, presentation, utensils, and behavioral/sensory techniques. The speech language pathologists work closely with the caregiver using videotapes, modeling, supervised guidance, and educational materials.

As our feeding program continues to grow and flourish, we continue to learn from our diverse population. In some instances, we have been able to replace standard feeding protocols with more innovative techniques such as "food chaining." These advancements in the evaluation and treatment of pediatric feeding disorders are the result of hard work and dedication. In this book, two of our speech pathologists, Cheri Fraker and Laura Walbert, will share their experiences with the reader and attempt to provide insight into these important issues.

I am lucky to be a part of this feeding team. Each case we treat is unique to that particular patient. As we continue treating children with eating problems we continue to learn. The goal is to have each child we treat not have life revolve around eating but to eat as a normal part of life.

Mark Fishbein, MD
Pediatric Gastroenterologist
SIU School of Medicine

How to Use This Book

This book was written to be a guide for evaluation and treatment of infants and children with feeding disorders. We formatted the book as a quick, yet extremely detailed, reference guide for the busy therapist with research from physicians to support the work that we do. Physician based research studies are italicized. "Chat sections" are included and that is our opportunity to talk directly to the reader about these subjects the way we do during our lectures. Each section has information that can be used either as a study guide for the student or new clinician or as a reference for evaluation and treatment by the experienced therapist.

We strongly believe that premature infants and children with complex medical issues carry their history with them throughout their lives and it shows particularly in the development of their feeding skills. In order to effectively treat these patients, the therapist needs an understanding of the child's medical history, detailed information regarding development of oral motor skills and the ability to develop the experience to truly see the child and recognize the complex motor, sensory and behavioral components that impact feeding. The therapist also must appreciate the complexity of selecting bottles, utensils and foods that meet the child's particular needs. We are not feeders, we make feedings therapeutic, we pick nipples, cups and spoons that will facilitate the development of the oral facial musculature. We position children so they have optimal respiratory function, physiological stability and control for safe and efficient swallowing.

The whole body approach to feeding is strongly recommended, we must outline our treatment accordingly. Find the factors in the child's history that are neurological in origin, explore the child's respiratory history and assess how that is impacting feeding and then ask questions regarding digestion to determine if the last phase of feeding has a negative or positive outcome for a child. Share this information with the child's physician. Infants and children who have pain or discomfort after eating will often have significant feeding problems.

As for content, evaluation of the swallow is discussed and aspiration management strategies are provided. In Chapter 11 a detailed multi-disciplinary intake and referral guide with red flag issues highlighted, is included to assist the therapist in the evaluation/treatment process for all feeding patients. The book contains a medical reference guide to help the therapist interpret the patient's medical history. Nutrition and digestive disorders are also outlined to help the therapist recognize symptoms to include in their report to the physician.

We tackle assessment and treatment from the NICU infant to childhood. Feeding skills are outlined by age of the child and there are references for appropriate volume of food per day. Meal and snack schedules are discussed as well as behavior management strategies. Our technique of "food chaining" is defined and demonstrated for the therapist to select appropriate foods for the treatment program. Selecting the right foods at the right time is critical to the treatment program. Breastfeeding assessment and treatment guidelines are also discussed to help make feeding successful for mother and baby and to recognize the special needs of the premature infant. There is also a comparison chart of all nipples on the market to help the therapist determine which nipple will best facilitate lip and cheek activation, tongue grooving, bolus formulation and control as well as provide the safest flow rate for the baby.

Treatment guidelines are detailed and there are sections in the book devoted to feeding aversion as well as special topics such as cerebral palsy, autism, gastroesophageal reflux, cleft lip/palate and tracheoesophageal fistula. We do not provide "cookbook" ideas for treatment, but guide the therapist through the process to find the core issues that impact feeding and expand the knowledge base to design a comprehensive, effective treatment program. We must caution the reader, that our book is in no way a substitute for the thorough and complete evaluation of feeding by an experienced feeding team or feeding specialist/speech pathologist.

Our program works from the idea of trying to step into the child's shoes and experience what they feel during feeding and finding fun, age appropriate, exciting methods of treatment. This project will always be a "work in progress" as we continually try to expand our knowledge base and our clinical skills. We hope that it meets the needs of therapists who are taking on the difficult, demanding, but extremely rewarding job of working with infants, children and families struggling with feeding problems.

Introduction

Everyone is an expert on feeding problems, so it seems. When children have difficulty feeding, the parents are bombarded with advice from family, friends and acquaintances as well as the medical community. Due to the complexity of pediatric feeding disorders, multi-disciplinary care is needed to identify the contributing factors and to determine the true heart of the disorder. Diagnosing a feeding disorder is like putting a large puzzle together.

Each piece of the puzzle is significant to treatment, but with most children there is the one core component or driving force behind the disorder. We should not accept easy answers or labels, such as, "nipple confusion" or "feeding aversion" or we will miss important information about the disorder and our treatment programs will not be complete. Nipple confusion can also be flow rate confusion or bottle/bottle confusion. The therapist needs to look carefully at these patients. With feeding aversion, what specifically is the child aversive to? Analyze accepted foods as well as rejected foods. Are there underlying physical problems that interfere with successful feeding? Children refuse to eat for a reason. Try to experience everything the child is experiencing, so you can start to put the pieces together.

What is needed is to become an expert on the individual child. We need to know his medical history, his past feeding history, his developmental level, his preferences, his oral motor skill level, his positioning needs and all the factors physical, emotional and social that shape his feeding behaviors. Treatment also extends beyond the child to the family and all caregivers. We need to analyze the feeding environment and the social-emotional relationships within the family. We need to do so with care and concern. Many families have faced extreme stress from high-risk pregnancies to the present feeding problems. These stresses impact the social situation and also the feeding relationship.

We encourage you to strive for excellence in your treatment programs and to give each child the care you would want for your own. We hope to provide some of the information necessary to provide comprehensive care for your patients and their families. Feeding therapy is difficult, draining and at times, very frustrating. The support of a team helps the therapists and provides the best care for the child and his family. If you do not have the benefit of working with a pediatric feeding team, we encourage you to network in your community to find professionals who can assist you in care of these challenging patients. We encourage you to pursue continuing education courses and literature to support you in your work. Many talented people have shared their knowledge, insight and talents with us and have helped us in our ongoing quest to continue to develop our skills and we are truly grateful for the experience.

Cheri and Laura

Why Feeding Therapy?
Ask the Doctor

Physician-based research studies are included for the therapist to share with medical staff and these references can also be used to justify treatment plans when dealing with insurance companies. Our physicians have requested journal articles addressing feeding therapy and these are some of the best articles we have found. Additional research excerpts from medical journals will be highlighted at the beginning of each chapter in the book or italicized in the text.

> *"Feeding disorders are common in early childhood, with the reported incidence of minor feeding problems ranging between 25% and 35 % in normal children and with more severe feeding problems observed in 40% to 70% in infants born prematurely or children with chronic medical conditions. Symptoms of feeding and swallowing disorders in children have many manifestations and clinical presentations including food refusal, failure to thrive, oral aversion, recurrent pneumonia, chronic lung disease or recurrent emesis. Anatomic or functional disorders that make feeding difficult or uncomfortable for the child may result in a learned aversion to eating, even after the underlying disorder is corrected. Delays in the initiation of feeding may affect the normal acquisition of feeding skills. The complexity of the feeding process and multiple interacting factors that affect the acquisition of feeding skills make the diagnosis and treatment of feeding disorders particularly challenging and complicated."*
>
> --Rudolph C, Link D: Feeding Disorders in Infants and Children. Pediatric Clinics of North America. Volume 49, number 1, February 2002.

> *"Observation of a feeding session by experienced occupational therapists, speech pathologists, psychologists, and nurses often provides tremendous insight into the underlying feeding problem. Positive interactions between the child and parent, such as shared eye contact, reciprocal vocalizations, praise and touch, or negative interactions, such as forced feeding, lack of conversation, eye contact or touch, threatening, bribing, and inconsistency are noted. Observations of the child's responses to offered foods, including disruptive behaviors, such as turning the head away from food or throwing of food, provide valuable information. These observations highlight primary or secondary behavior problems that allow for future structuring of appropriate behavior treatment interventions."*
>
> --Rudolph C, Link D: Feeding Disorders in Infants and Children. Pediatric Clinics of North America. Volume 49, number 1, February 2002.

"A study of children with special health care needs in Washington State found that nutrition or feeding-team intervention for disabled children who had slow growth or failure to thrive improved dietary intake and adequacy in all of the children who had inappropriate or inadequate intake, decreased illness and hospitalization, improved feeding skills, improved feeding behavior, decreased constipation, and enhanced developmental feeding progress. Estimated medical cost savings achieved by providing nutritional or feeding team services ranged from $180 to $5000 per year, per child. Optimally, the team should include the disciplines of speech pathology, occupational therapy, psychology, nutrition, gastroenterology, and otolaryngology for the core evaluation. Support from other specialists in radiology, social services, child life, neurology, and pulmonary medicine often is used. An interdisciplinary evaluation facilitates integration of expertise from different disciplines to provide insight into the various factors that interact in contributing to the child's swallowing disorder and overall health."

> --Lucas B, Nardella M, Feucht S: Cost considerations: The benefits of nutrition services for a case series of children with special health care needs in Washington State. Dev Iss 17:1-4, 1999.

"A child may refuse to eat even after an underlying anatomic abnormality has been corrected due to a learned aversion to feeding. Behavior therapy often can overcome this type of "conditioned" food refusal. Various therapeutic approaches may improve the efficiency and safety of feeding. These include changing the texture of foods, pacing of the feeding, changing the bottle or utensils; and changing the alignment of the head, neck, and body with feeding. One small study showed that the systematic presentation of food in a consistent manner improved feeding skills in some children even with neurologic impairments."

> --Babbitt RL, et al: Behavioral assessment and treatment of pediatric feeding disorders. J Dev Behav Pediatr 15:278-291, 1994

"In children with developmental disabilities, diagnosis-specific treatment of feeding disorders results in significantly improved energy consumption and nutritional status. These data also indicate that decreased morbidity (reflected by a lower acute care hospitalization rate) may be related, at least in part, to successful management of feeding problems. Our results emphasize the importance of a structured approach to these problems, and we propose a diagnostic and treatment algorithm for children with developmental disabilities and suspected feeding disorders. Children with developmental disabilities are at increased risk for developing feeding-related difficulties, including gastroesophageal reflux, oral motor dysfunction, pharyngoesophageal dyskinesia, and aversive feeding behavior. If not adequately treated, feeding disorders may result in additional complications including esophagitis, reactive airway disease, aspiration pneumonia, and bedsores. Previous reports indicate that enteral feeding regimens for nutrition support in developmentally disabled children improve overall nutritional status."

> --Schwarz S, Corredor J, Fisher-Medina J, Cohen J, Rabinowitz S: Diagnosis and Treatment of Feeding Disorders in Children with Developmental Disabilities. Pediatrics Vol 108, Number 3, Sept 2001.

"At each stage of development, the infant nervous system is primed to acquire new motor skills. A lack of feeding experience during these "critical periods" of development results in great difficulty mastering the skills later in life; infants may not be able to eat orally for the first months of life may learn how to spoon- and cup-feed without ever learning an effective nutritive suck and swallow. Development of the oral phase requires normal anatomy, intact sensory feedback, and normal muscle strength and coordination. Children with neuromuscular disorders often present initially with poor feeding skills in infancy."

> --Rudolph C, Link D: Feeding Disorders in Infants and Children. Pediatric Clinics of North America. Volume 49, number 1, February 2002.

"Specific feeding aversions have been observed in children after cancer chemotherapy and in children with metabolic disorders that result in discomfort after ingestions of specific foods. More generalized feeding aversions develop if an infant aspirates or chokes during feeding or experiences pain in temporal proximity to feeding. Infants who have experienced prolonged airway intubation or tube feeding often have learned that any efforts to approach their mouth or face will result in discomfort from airway suctioning, tape removal, or tube manipulation. Therefore they resist efforts to approach their mouths. When they are able to eat, this "oral aversion" must be gently extinguished."

> --Rudolph C: Feeding Disorders in Infants and Children. Journal of Pediatrics 1994;125:S116-24

CHAPTER ONE

▲

Swallowing

What's Up, Doc?

The following medical journal excerpts are included for the therapist to share with physicians. Our physicians have asked us for physician-based research on feeding therapy, infant swallowing and modified barium swallow studies. We feel these articles will be useful to other therapists working in high-risk nurseries and pediatric units, so we included them at the beginning of chapters for a quick and easy reference.

"Coordination of the oral and pharyngeal phases of swallowing is essential for prevention of aspiration. During swallowing, respiration ceases and the pharynx is cleared before respiration resumes. If either of these protective mechanisms fails, aspiration of milk can occur despite anatomic protection. If there is a lack of relaxation of the upper esophageal sphincter (cricopharyngeal achalasia) the pharynx will not be cleared and aspiration may result. Similarly, if inspiration occurs during the swallow, aspiration may result. Coordination of swallowing and breathing is particularly challenging in the infant in whom the respiratory rate is relatively high. During vigorous sucking and swallowing, as occurs early in a feeding session, there is often a significant reduction in minute ventilation with mild hypoxia, even in normal infants; patients with compromised cardiac or respiratory function often have serious difficulties with hypoxia during the feeding. In the preterm infant, the coordination of sucking, swallowing and breathing is not fully mature. Preterm infants tend to hold their breath for several seconds, during which time a number of sucks and swallows occur. This pattern of multiple swallows without respiration decreases with increasing postconceptual age."
>   *--Hanlon MB, et al: Deglutition apnea as indicator of maturation of suckle feeding in bottle-fed preterm infants. Dev Med Child Neurol 39:534-542, 1997*

"Any patient with aspiration in addition to a significant feeding disorder with clinical findings suggestive of cranial nerve IX or X involvement should undergo MR imaging to diagnose brain stem, skull base, or spinal problems that can interfere with swallowing, such as a Chiari malformation. MR imaging of the chest is useful in patients suspected of having a vascular ring/sling cause for stridor or dysphagia. Chest CT scanning may be particularly useful to assess the severity or progression of chronic pulmonary disease, which affects decisions regarding feeding safety. GI endoscopy may be useful in selected cases to rule out strictures, webs, or inflammatory lesions definitively in the esophagus and stomach, but it is generally not a substitute for radiologic evaluation."
>   *--Rudolph C, Link D: Feeding Disorders in Infants and Children. Pediatric Clinics of North America. Volume 49, number 1, February 2002*

Therapist to Therapist

Evaluation of the swallow is the single most challenging aspect of feeding therapy. Children with complex medical histories may present with different symptoms day to day. These children are variable due to tone, fatigue and respiratory or digestive tract issues. Therefore, procedures and observations should be completed over several therapy sessions to get accurate information and a true feel for the child's feeding capabilities. Then, once in treatment, the high-risk or medically fragile patient's swallow warrants frequent re-assessment to monitor change or improvement. There are procedures to assess the swallow, modified barium swallow studies and FEES (see Chapter Two) that reflect the presence (or absence) of momentary aspiration. These valuable studies are crucial to the thorough evaluation of feeding capability and skills; however, the studies have limitations and must be completed correctly.

Structure the evaluation session to gather maximum information possible about the patient. First of all, have the parent participate. The parent can provide the therapist with a wealth of information about their child. They often can very accurately describe their child's feeding disorder if given the chance to discuss it at length. Feeding a child is a reciprocal act. You must evaluate both the child and the feeder to observe the feeding relationship. Ask the parent to feed the child during the evaluation or via videotape at home, so you can observe the techniques used, the amount of food placed in the mouth and the rate of feeding. Watch for potential aspiration. We have evaluated many children who aspirate because food was placed too deeply into the mouth or the pace of the meal was too fast and the child simply could not adequately clear the pharynx in one swallow. However, there are also very complex, multi-factoral cases of dysphagia where there are no simple answers and treatment is extremely challenging. Team intervention is essential, especially when working with these children.

We feel the use of cervical auscultation (stethoscope to the side of the neck) can be very beneficial during the swallowing evaluation. Cervical auscultation helps the therapist monitor the pharyngeal stage of the swallow. We have found that the more we use cervical auscultation, the more we rely on it. However, do know that cervical auscultation does not replace modified barium studies or FEES. In fact, silent aspiration can be easily missed with cervical auscultation. The silent aspiration case is the most difficult, as some children show no outward sign of a problem with swallowing or have not yet presented with a significant illness.

When evaluating the actual act of swallowing, look closely at the stages and write down what you see. Begin problem solving. Literally take the swallow apart phase by phase and mimic, in your own mouth, what the child is doing. This will help you to feel what is happening and to start developing your treatment plan.

Ask Yourself These Questions

SECRETION MANAGEMENT

As you listen with your stethoscope before the feeding, are secretions pooling in the pharynx? Is the child having significant problems managing saliva? How difficult is it to manage a bolus with a large amount of saliva already present in the mouth? Do you need to write a saliva management program as the first step in your treatment approach?

APPETITE

How does the child react when food is introduced? Does he open his mouth or turn away? Does he seem hungry? Is feeding a pleasant experience?

BOLUS FORMATION AND CONTROL

When food is in the mouth, where does it go? Is the bolus on the middle of the tongue, in the lateral sulci of the cheeks or is it falling back prematurely into the pharynx? Time the oral stage; does food remain in the mouth too long or does the child swallow without chewing?

NEUROLOGICAL CONCERNS

Does the infant have a tonic bite reflex or excessive tremor in the tongue? Can the child maintain state of alertness and organization? Is the child arching? Are the oral reflexes intact?

Add the cranial nerve assessment to your evaluation. It can become an integral part of your evaluation. This is information that is valuable to therapists and physicians. We have the opportunity to evaluate cranial nerve function during a meal. This information will assist the team in deciding if a consult with a pediatric neurologist is indicated. We can share information with the physician about the child's response to taste and the movement and control of the structures, especially the tongue. (Please refer to the *Swallowing and the Nervous System* section in this chapter.)

ORAL STRUCTURES AND FUNCTION

Can the child close his mouth completely? Are the lips sealed and cheeks active so there is adequate negative pressure and force to provide the push to help move food back for swallowing?

What does the tongue look like? Where is it at rest? Is there a central groove? Can the child form a bolus? Is the tongue strong enough to propel the bolus posteriorly?

When the swallow triggers, does the child sound clear afterward? Does a second swallow help? Does the child need several swallows to clear the pharynx? Remember, cervical auscultation is a great tool to monitor a child session to session, but it is not a guarantee of clear swallows or a replacement for a MBS (Modified Barium Swallow) or FEES (Fiberoptic Endoscopic Evaluation of Swallowing) assessment. A stethoscope does not pick up silent aspiration. If you have concerns, a complete evaluation is warranted.

POSITIONING

Is the positioning of the patient conducive to good feeding function? Is the position of the head and neck appropriate? Would a slight or major modification help? As a brief note, be cautious in changing the feeding position of children with cerebral palsy too quickly. They have a system of sensory feedback that they rely on to eat and when their position is changed suddenly, they may aspirate. Modify their positioning slowly and appropriately with the guidance of the occupational and/or physical therapist.

GI CONCERNS

Is gastroesophageal reflux an issue? Is the child experiencing *gastropharyngeal* reflux and coughing because of the backflow of gastric content into the pharynx?

How far apart are the feedings? Is there adequate time for digestion? Is the child receiving adequate nutrition to have the strength to eat? Or is the child fed so frequently that reflux and gastric discomfort are creating an aversion?

Is constipation impacting the child's comfort level and desire to eat? Children with cerebral palsy often have problems with constipation and this can dramatically impact oral intake. Does the child have recurrent diarrhea after eating? Are there concerns about malabsorption? Share your findings and feeding observations with the physician or pediatric gastroenterologist. (Refer to Chapter 10 for information regarding digestive tract disorders.)

FEEDING METHOD

With infants, what nipple is the baby using? Some infants are fed with four or five different brands of bottles. The texture, firmness and flow rate of market brand nipples varies significantly. It is extremely important to have the right nipple for treatment. (Refer to Chapter 11 for nipple comparison chart and detailed information about the right products for feeding.) For older children, analyze the appropriateness of the cups and utensils, and how are they affecting the child's feedings. Would a change be beneficial?

Is the family mixing the formula correctly? Is the formula right for the baby's needs? Does the family use the same formula consistently or purchase what is on sale week to week?

Is the mother breastfeeding? Does she have an adequate milk supply or over-active let down? Can the baby keep up with the flow rate? Is latch-on correct? Can position change help mother and baby have a successful breastfeeding experience?

APPETITE RECOMMENDATIONS AND REFERRALS

Write treatment program goals in the chart as part of your evaluation note. Inform the doctor and the family as to what the baby is doing at the present time and what your initial plan of treatment involves. We often write 24-48 hour initial treatment goals and post them bedside in the NICU. This helps all nursing shifts be aware of the treatment plan and staff will not be as easily tempted to make a change if they are aware of the program goals.

Give the staff a way to communicate concerns to you easily and directly. We often put bright neon colored communication logs on the patient's clipboard. We have our initial goals printed on the sheet and we also ask for suggestions and concerns from nursing staff. This gives the therapist a great deal of information from night and evening shift staff and these observations can help in the diagnostic process.

Swallowing

Swallowing therapy is stressful, time consuming and a very complex process. Protect yourself as the feeding professional. If a doctor, for example, expresses reluctance in allowing you to assess the swallow comprehensively, be persistent in your procedures and recommendations and back up your concerns with observations, facts, physician-based research and documentation. Many times, the physician simply requires additional information about the study and the information it can provide. Remember, it is your name on the report, you have an obligation to advocate for your patient. You may have to push for a modified barium swallow or FEES test, but these tools are part of our evaluation process. Be confident in your recommendations!

Suggestions for Therapy

To initiate our venture into therapy techniques, following are several specific treatment options that may help you address a variety of swallowing difficulties and issues.

NIPPLE TYPE, SIZE AND FLOW RATE

What nipple is being used? Refer to the Nipple Comparison Chart (in Chapter 11). The flow rate varies from nipple to nipple and cup to cup. Each brand is different and can dramatically affect swallowing safety. Questions to ask: Did the parent cut the nipple to get thickened feedings through? Is the feeding is too thick? With thickened feedings, try a high flow nipple, such as, a Gerber fast flow silicone nipple, or a Dr. Brown Y-cut nipple. Avoid crosscut nipples that can shoot liquid into the pharynx prematurely. Some infa-feeder nipples are so large, the child cannot form or control the bolus of pureed food and it may fall prematurely into the pharynx. Repetitive sucking of thick consistency liquid puree may pose a hazard due to the ongoing coating of the posterior pharynx.

BOLUS SIZE

Reduce the size of the bolus for easier manipulation and swallowing. What type of spoon is used to feed the child?

FOOD CHARACTERISTICS

Assess the foods you are using with the child. Do the selected foods coat the throat or clear easily? For example, mashed potatoes coat the throat; applesauce clears easily. Ice cream coats the throat; orange sherbet clears easily. Alternating food consistencies may help the child clear the pharynx easier.

COLD FOOD AND LIQUID

Use very cold liquid and/or food as thermal stimulation to call attention to the mouth and generate muscle contraction. If the patient has cardiac issues, consult the physician prior to utilizing this technique.

5

FLAVOR AND CARBONATION

Use strong flavor and carbonation in the liquids to intensify the sensory input. This may improve the triggering of the swallow.

ANALYZING AND POSITIONING AND FUNCTIONS

Look carefully at the child's trunk, head and extremities. Is the body well supported? Is his breathing appropriate? Is he postured so as to reduce pressure on the stomach while eating and possibly decreasing the risk of gastropharyngeal reflux after the feeding? Are the shoulders down or high around the neck? Is there adequate support to the pelvis and feet? Note laryngeal elevation when the position of the jaw is modified slightly. Consult with an occupational therapist (OT) and/or physical therapist (PT). Take photos of the child's optimal body/head positioning. Photographs can be used for a positioning guide for other professionals and caregivers involved in the child's feeding program.

MANIPULATING ORAL-FACIAL MUSCLES

If muscles of the lips, cheeks and tongue have some incapabilities, apply massage (sensory assistance) or support to the jaw (stabilization assistance). When applying stabilization assistance, avoid applying too much pressure. The goal is to offer support, not inhibit movement and generate resistance. Also, avoid inhibiting the "floor" muscles of the tongue by pushing under the chin; make sure jaw support is directly on the mandible.

▲

Work with the child, modify what you can, and train the feeders. Alter positioning, food types, utensils and bottles as needed and if concerns persist, follow-up with additional evaluations. Diagnostic therapy is indicated with many children with swallow dysfunction. Interpret any changes in respiratory status as a red flag. Also note that children with muscle tone issues may also be affected by growth. As the body grows and changes, gravity will continue to affect the body and the swallow in new ways. Watch and observe, and listen to the voice within you. If your concerns persist, encourage a complete re-evaluation.

Emily: Aspiration Case Study

HISTORY

Emily was a term infant who was transferred to NICU following delivery at a local hospital. Emily was stressed during delivery and passed meconium in the amniotic fluid. She did not aspirate the meconium, but she was in respiratory distress and was intubated before she was transferred to the neonatal intensive care unit. When Emily arrived at the hospital, the staff noted that she was intubated with a tube that was quite large for an infant her size. A nasogastric tube was used to give Emily her feedings. Although Emily responded well to treatment and was soon was well enough to start oral feeding attempts, she coughed and choked on the bottle and did not appear to be able to swallow efficiently. The nursing staff also reported stridor (audible breathing) and speech therapy was consulted to evaluate the swallow and treat as needed.

EVALUATION FINDINGS

The speech therapist completed the bedside evaluation of the swallow. Root, suck, phasic bite and transverse tongue reflexes were intact. The gag reflex was absent. Secretion swallow was weak and very difficult to detect via cervical auscultation. A consult with the otolaryngologist, also known as the ear, nose and throat physician (ENT), and a modified barium swallow study were recommended by the therapist and completed the same day.

The otolaryngologist reported swelling in the pharynx. The modified barium swallow study revealed silent aspiration with significantly decreased laryngeal elevation.

The therapist, physicians and the radiologist viewed the tape of the MBS together several times, frame by frame. The team discussed the findings and the physician suspected laryngeal trauma due to the size of the intubation tube used at the local hospital. The speech therapist agreed that Emily needed time for swelling to go down, but was concerned regarding the silent aspiration. No cough triggered, her eyes did not water and she showed no visible signs of aspiration.

It was felt direct swallow stimulation should continue daily. It was assumed that Emily was not feeling the formula in her throat as her pharyngeal receptors did not appear to be responding when she aspirated formula. The speech therapist started a thermal swallow stimulation program with ice-cold formula given in single swallows via syringe while Emily was actively sucking on her pacifier. The single bolus was given and followed by assisted jaw closure and an occasional light stroke down the throat to encourage swallowing. Thermal stimulation was completed for a few minutes, six times per day.

The parents were initially trained to dip Emily's pacifier in cold formula and the speech therapist met with them every day to complete training and answer questions about their daughter. Emily's parents fully supported the treatment plan and were soon independently completing thermal stimulation sessions using the pacifier and syringe. Cervical auscultation was used to monitor the swallow daily. Emily was placed in a side-tilt position to allow formula to collect briefly in the cheek prior to entering the pharynx. This position mimics the position of infants who are breastfed. The parents were instructed how to position their daughter for therapeutic tastes and were told that this technique would allow increased bolus control and would help reduce the risk of premature spillage of liquid into the pharynx.

Toward the end of the week, the speech therapist gave Emily successive cold swallows with pacifier and syringe and then moved to 3 cc's cold formula in a bottle and imposed breaks as needed.

A follow-up modified barium swallow study was completed one week later to assess swallowing improvement. The second swallow evaluation was completed without the NG tube in place. There was no aspiration when Emily took her first ounce of chilled formula. Laryngeal elevation was improved but still significantly reduced. Due to the increasing loss of coordination toward the end of the first 30 cc's, the speech therapist and radiologist decided to continue to evaluate the swallow for the second ounce (with a trial of warm formula and barium feeding). Emily silently aspirated as the second ounce of formula was introduced.

The physician also viewed the study and the pediatric gastroenterologist was consulted as there was a possibility that Emily would require a g-tube. Emily was re-evaluated by the otolaryngologist who reported less stridor and some reduction of the swelling in the pharynx. The team decided that the best course of treatment would be to place a silastic feeding tube (soft nasogastric tube that can remain in place for several weeks before changing) for a two-week period and allow Emily to be discharged from the hospital. Emily was transferred to the care of the pediatric feeding team as an outpatient with home nursing and continued consultation from the pediatric gastroenterologist and speech therapist. The daily thermal stimulation program was continued. Thermal stimulation now consisted of 5-10 cc feedings of chilled formula using a Gerber medium flow nipple on a Munchkin Medicator Cup. The medicator cup holds only 10 cc's of liquid and was used to limit the amount given orally. The third modified barium was scheduled for completion after two additional weeks of treatment. The therapist recommended that the silastic tube be removed by home nursing service at least four hours prior to the final modified barium swallow study.

RESULTS

The third swallow evaluation was completed and the team again carefully assessed the swallow with room temperature formula and barium. There were no signs of aspiration or laryngeal penetration. Emily's feedings were assessed several times that month by the speech therapist and the family was advised to contact the team immediately if they had any new concerns regarding feedings. Follow-up visits were scheduled with the otolaryngologist and pediatric gastroenterologist. Emily did well and displayed no additional feeding difficulties.

The Swallowing Sequence

The following information is a review of the swallow and what occurs at each stage of swallowing. Several descriptions from different authors are provided for the therapist. A cranial nerve assessment is also provided to assist in the diagnostic process. Many physicians will request information regarding cranial nerve function when a patient presents with swallow dysfunction. We often share Dr. Colin Rudolph's description of swallowing phases with our residents and physicians. We use that information to as a guide to discuss the treatment plan or to express why we feel a modified barium swallow study is necessary.

Swallowing and the Nervous System

NEURAL CONTROL OF SWALLOWING

According to Dodds, 1989, Dodds, Stewart, and Logemann 1990, there are four major components involved in the neural control of swallowing. These include:
1. Afferent sensory fibers contained in the cranial nerves,
2. Cerebral, midbrain and cerebeller fibers that synapse with the brainstem swallowing centers,
3. Paired swallowing centers in the brainstem, and
4. Efferent motor fibers contained in the cranial nerves.

CRANIAL NERVE ASSESSMENT

	Cranial Nerve	*Bedside Testing Mechanism*
I.	Olfactory	Place ammonia under the nose, response is startle or grimace
II.	Optic	Check PERL (pupils equal and reactive to light)
III.	Oculomotor	PERL, EOM (extraocular movements) full and conjugate
IV.	Trochlear	Same testing mechanism as oculomotor
V.	Trigeminal	Touch cheek; infant should turn toward stimulus
VI.	Abducens	Rotate infant; eyes look in direction of travel
VII.	Facial	Asymmetrical facial movements
VIII.	Auditory	Infant quiets to voice, blinks to clap of hands
IX.	Glossopharyngeal	Strong gag response
X.	Vagus	Cry is not hoarse
XI.	Accessory	Turn supine infant's head to one side; infant attempts to bring head to midline
XII.	Hypoglossal	Insert finger in mouth while sucking; note force of tongue; note vesiculations or quivering tongue

Oral Reflexes Present in the Term Infant

(Referenced from Arvedson and Brodsky.)

Reflex	*Stimulus*	*Cranial Nerves*
Root	Touch corner of mouth Or pull down the lower lip	V, VII, XI, XII
Gag	Touch posterior tongue Persists	IX, X
Phasic Bite	Pressure on gums	V
Tongue Protrusion	Touch to tongue or lips	XII
Transverse Tongue Suckling	Nipple in mouth	V, VII, IX, XII
Swallowing	Bolus of food in pharynx	V, VII, IX, X, XII

Cranial Nerve Function

If you are working with an infant or child who demonstrates signs of cranial nerve dysfunction, recommend a consultation with a pediatric neurologist.

TRIGEMINAL

The trigeminal nerve arises within the pons and travels to the jaw muscles. It powers chewing, soft palate movement for sucking, and initiation of swallowing. The sensory component provides proprioceptive input of the temporal mandibular joint, tongue and palate, and sensory feedback for sucking.
If cranial nerve deficits are present the following may be observed:

- Immature, or poorly coordinated, or absent movement of the mandible
- The presence of a jaw jerk reflex (exaggerated or absent), and
- The presence of a tonic bite reflex.

FACIAL NERVE

The facial nerve also arises in the pons and innervates the muscles of facial expression, the eyelids and muscles of mastication. It is involved in secretion control. Its fibers bring taste sensation from the anterior two-thirds of the tongue back to the brain stem. The facial nerve also influences rooting, sucking and swallowing.
Cranial nerve deficits may result in:

- Paralysis of the lower half of the face
- Unilateral or bilateral paralysis, and
- Paralysis of the forehead.

GLOSSOPHARYNGEAL

The glossopharyngeal nerve has both sensory and motor fibers. It brings sensation from the larynx and pharynx, sends motor nerve fibers to the throat to power swallowing and is partially responsible for initiation of a gag reflex. Its fibers bring taste sensation from the posterior one-third of the tongue back to the brain stem.
If cranial nerve deficits are present the following may be observed:

- Weakness or asymmetry of the muscular palate
- Flattening of the palatopharyngeal folds, or
- Vocal fold paralysis.

VAGAL NERVE

The vagal nerve is a mixed nerve that has motor fibers that come from the medulla. This nerve is involved in swallowing and regulation of cardiac, pulmonary, and part of gastrointestinal function. It brings sensation from the gastro-intestinal (GI) tract back to the medulla. It innervates muscles of the palate, uvula, palatal arches, pharynx, vocal folds as well as the swallow, respiration and digestive functions. Sensory components of this nerve include taste from base of tongue and palate and additional sensory information from the pharynx, larynx, trachea, lungs, tongue, bronchi and heart.

HYPOGLOSSAL NERVE

The hypoglossal nerve is involved with the complex movements of the tongue, hyoid and larynx, which are all important components of swallowing.
If deficits are present you may observe:

- Tongue movements that are dysfunctional
- Exaggerated tongue protrusion
- Unilateral or bilateral absence of tongue movement
- Tongue fasiculations, or
- Tongue atrophy.

The Suck-Swallow-Breathe Sequence

THE FIRST STAGE

The first stage of swallowing is voluntary, where the bolus is pushed from the mouth into the oropharynx mainly by the movements of the tongue. The tongue is raised and pressed against the hard palate by the intrinsic muscles of the tongue.

THE SECOND STAGE

The second stage of swallowing is involuntary and is usually very rapid. It involves contraction of the walls of the pharynx. Breathing and chewing stop and successive contractions of the three constrictor muscles move the food through the oral and laryngeal parts of the pharynx. The bolus of food is prevented from entering the nasopharynx by elevation of the soft palate. The tensor veli palatini and levator veli palatini muscles tense and elevate the soft palate against the posterior wall of the pharynx. These actions close the pharyngeal isthmus, thereby preventing food from entering the nasopharynx.
As the bolus passes through the oropharynx, the walls of the pharynx are raised. The contraction of the phayrngeal muscles elevates the pharynx and the larynx. The palatopharyngeus and stylopharyngeus muscles elevate the larynx and pharynx in swallowing. The hyoid bone is raised and fixed during swallowing by contraction of the geniohyoid, mylohyoid, digastric and stylohyoid muscles.
During swallowing the vestibule of the larynx is closed, the epiglottis is bent posteriorly over the inlet of the larynx and the aryepiglottic folds are approximated. These folds provide lateral food channels that guide the bolus of food from the sides of the epiglottis and the closed inlet of the larynx. All those actions are designed to prevent food from entering the larynx.

THE THIRD STAGE

The third stage of swallowing squeezes the bolus from the laryngopharynx into the esophagus. This wave is produced by the inferior constrictor muscle of the pharynx. The food is passed through the esophagus to the stomach.

Phases of Deglutition

Logemann, 1998 describes four phases of deglutition:
1. The Oral Preparatory Phase
2. The Oral Phase
3. The Pharyngeal Phase, and
4. The Esophageal Phase.

Each phase is important in accomplishing an efficient and effective swallow. The following describes each phase, and how a disordered swallow can impact successful deglutition. These descriptions may also be used for writing detailed reports for physicians or for developing the child's treatment program.

1. ORAL PREPARATORY PHASE

The oral preparatory phase is described as the stage of sensory recognition of the food as it approaches the mouth and the oral manipulation that occurs to hold and form the bolus. The larynx and pharynx are at rest, the airway is open and nasal breathing continues. Dysphagia results if a child loses control of the bolus and material falls into an open airway. The cause of this occurring may result from:

- Reduced lip closure
- Reduced tongue shaping and/or coordination
- Reduced tongue motion or coordination
- Reduced labial tension
- Reduced buccal tension
- Reduced tongue control

2. ORAL PHASE

The oral phase includes food manipulation or mastication and the act of the tongue propeling the food posteriorly. Dysphagia results if any of the following is disordered:

- Delayed oral onset-of-swallow secondary to apraxia of swallow or reduced oral sensation
- Apraxia of the swallow
- Tongue thrust
- Reduced labial tension and/or tone
- Reduced buccal tension and/or tone
- Reduced tongue strength
- Reduced tongue elevation

Swallowing

- Reduced anterior-posterior tongue movement
- Reduced tongue control

3. PHARYNGEAL PHASE

The pharyngeal phase begins with the triggering of the pharyngeal swallow. The triggering of the swallow results in elevation and retraction of the velum, elevation and anterior movement of the hyoid and larynx, closure of the larynx, opening of the cricopharyngeal sphincter, ramping of the base of tongue, and top down peristalsis of the pharyngeal constrictors. Dysphagia results if any of the following occur:

- Reduced velopharyngeal closure
- Reduced tongue base
- Reduced laryngeal elevation
- Delayed triggering of the pharyngeal swallow
- Reduced laryngeal closure at the level of the true folds, arytenoids to base of epiglottis and false folds, aryepiglottic folds and epiglottis
- Reduced posterior movement of the base of tongue

4. ESOPHAGEAL PHASE

The esophageal phase commences with the lowering of the larynx and the contraction of the cricopharyngeus. Normal esophageal transit time varies from 8 to 20 seconds. Some of the disorders of this phase of the swallow include:

- Esophageal backflow
- Tracheoesophageal fistula, and
- Zenker's diverticulum (pouch or pocket above the cricopharyngeal sphincter and associated with abnormal coordination of muscles in this area).

Feeding by Phase (Colin Rudolph, MD)

ORAL PHASE

To achieve an effective and efficient swallow during the oral phase of feeding, the following must occur: adequate sensory feedback from the mouth (cranial nerves V, VII, IX, X), intact strength and coordination of the orbicularis oris and buccal muscles (VII), appropriate function of the muscles of mastication (V) and the tongue (XII).

PHARYNGEAL PHASE

For infants, in the pharyngeal stage of swallowing, the larynx is high in the neck at C1 or C3 during respiration and the epiglottis almost passes up behind the soft palate, separating the respiratory and digestive tracts. Liquids then flow over the tongue, around the epiglottis into the isthmus faucium, through the pyriform sinuses, and into the esophagus.

The tongue lies entirely in the oral cavity. The elevated position of the larynx results in there being essentially no region where the airway and digestive tract cross. During the first 2 years of life, the larynx remains high in the neck, the first major descent occurs between 2 and 3 years of age as the upper border of the larynx descends to the level of C3 and the lower border to C5.

The larynx drops and prevents the epiglottis from approximating the soft palate. In the mature adult, even during maximum laryngeal elevation a region of the oropharynx is always located above the laryngeal inlet increasing the risk of aspiration during swallowing.

Pharyngeal swallows are initiated in response to stimulation by food or secretions in the pharynx. If the child has impaired sensation in the pharynx the risk of aspiration increases significantly. The upper pharynx and the soft palate close against the posterior pharynx, sealing the nasal cavity as the tongue propels the bolus into the phayrnx.

Respiration stops and the larynx is pulled up and forward by the mylohyoid, geniohyoid, and thyrohyoid muscles, moving the laryngeal inlet out of the path of the bolus. The larynx closes with the epiglottis flipping over the top of the larynx. Closure of the false and true folds also protects the laryngeal inlet. The upper esophageal sphincter opens and wave-like contraction of the pharyngeal constrictor muscles against the back surface of the tongue moves the bolus through the pharynx, past the lifted, closed layrnx and into the esophagus.

ESOPHAGEAL PHASE

The upper esophageal sphincter then relaxes to open and allows the food to pass into the esophagus. The peristaltic wave is dependent on information from vagal afferents. Proprioceptive input by cranial nerves (V, IX and X) then adjusts the peristaltic activity appropriately for different food sizes and consistencies.

In the esophageal stage, abnormal peristalsis, inflammation or esophageal atresia, stenosis, webs, vascular rings, tumor or foreign body may result in dysphagia in children. These problems are diagnosed by radiographic contrast examination or flexible endoscopy.

GASTROINTESTINAL AND ABSORPTIVE PHASE

Gastrointestinal and absorptive phase of feeding primarily results in positive or negative reinforcement of feeding. Problems during this stage of feeding include gastric distention from gastroparesis, dumping syndrome (common after fundoplication) or peptic disease associated with decreased appetite or food refusal or malabsorption problems, which can falsely trigger satiety.

CHAPTER TWO

Aspiration

"Laryngeal penetration is a benign, normal process in infants likely due to immaturity of the swallowing mechanism. It is not a reliable predictor of aspiration as it is in adults."
--(Delzell PB; Kraus RA; Gaisie G; Lerner GE, Laryngeal Penetration: A Predictor of Aspiration in Infants? Pediatric Radiology October 1999; 29(10): 762-5

"Swallowing dysfunction with aspiration is a common cause of feeding-related difficulties in childhood. In infants with feeding difficulties, a modified barium swallow study may demonstrate aspiration when the UGI is negative."
--Vazquez JL; Buonomo C, Feeding Difficulties in the first days of life: Findings on Upper Gastrointestinal Series and the Role of Videofluroscopic Swallowing Study. Pediatr Radiol-01-Dec-1999;29(12): 894-6

Aspiration in Infants and Children: Definitions and Risk Factors

Chronic aspiration can be detrimental to the patient and is one of the most important concerns when working with a child in feeding therapy. In addition to aspiration, there are several other factors of concern that can potentially occur during the abnormal swallowing process. Following are some useful definitions and supporting information.

When eating, the term *residue* is used to define the presence of un-cleared food left behind in the mouth or pharynx after the swallow. The terms *backflow* and *reflux* describe the act of food entering into the pharynx from the esophagus, or food entering into the nasal cavity from the oral cavity. When food or liquid enters into the larynx down to, but not below the true vocal cords the term *penetration* classifies this behavior. Though research studies suggest that laryngeal penetration is a normal process in infants, premature or medically fragile patients should be closely monitored if penetration is observed during a modified barium swallow study. These children often exhibit other risk factors that can place them at high risk for aspiration.

ASPIRATION

Aspiration is the entry of food or liquid into the airway that occurs below the level of the true vocal folds. Interestingly, some studies estimate that our lungs can handle aspiration of approximately 10-20% of what we swallow. While it is common for infants and children to aspirate in very small amounts when learning to eat, aspiration becomes problematic or can lead to pneumonia when patients consistently aspirate each time they swallow or aspirate periodically in larger amounts.

Respiratory Illness and Affect of Aspiration on Lung Tissue

During assessment, take care to note any former respiratory infections or signs of reflux, even in the absence of pneumonia. Frequent colds or respiratory infections can be significant indicators in determining possible aspiration. Keep in mind that if pneumonia has occurred in the past, the infant or child may have aspirated for a significant time prior to the resulting pneumonia. Vazquez and Buonomo contend that, *"neurologically normal children with GER (gastroesophageal reflux) are also at an increased risk of aspiration and may present with significant respiratory symptoms."*

Chronic undiagnosed aspiration can cause a build up of scar tissue in the lungs that can result in difficulty recovering from future upper respiratory illness or pneumonia. More is covered on this important subject in the next section *Aspiration and the Lungs.*

Vazquez and Buonomo continue, *"Aspiration occurs in children [who have] some type of local anatomic abnormalities that are acquired due to local trauma or infection or with some form of CNS dysfunction."* However, they add, silent aspiration can also occur in healthy infants with the following chronic or temporary symptoms: wheeze, stridor, cough, recurrent pneumonia, and apnea. *"The cause of these dysfunctions is unclear. They may have a form of delayed neuromuscular incoordination. These children should be closely monitored and a neurological evaluation should be done,"* according to Vazques and Buonomo.

Aspiration in Premature and Neurologically Impaired Children

Aspiration can also manifest in newborn infants, especially premature infants who lack the ability to coordinate their sucking, swallowing and breathing. By 34 weeks of gestational age, most premature infants are starting to be able to perform these suck-swallow-breath functions and begin bottle-feeding or attempts at breast-feeding. The maturation of oral and pharyngeal anatomy and the evolution of the suck-swallow-breath process develop parallel to the development of the brain and nervous system. When this developmental process falters, gagging, regurgitation, or choking may occur during feeding. When this happens the child is at risk and may fail to thrive. Recurrent respiratory infections and wheezing might accompany the feeding problems.

Neurologically impaired children are also at high risk for aspiration. They lack the maturation of neuromuscular coordination of the oral and pharyngeal muscles, which is complicated by the increased prevalence of gastroesophageal reflux. This is supported by Link, *"Laryngopharyngeal sensory deficits from neurologic disorders or decreased laryngeal sensitivity from chronic gastrolaryngeal reflux may predispose to problems with coordinating swallowing and increase aspiration risk."*

Infants with tachypnea (respiratory rate greater than 60 bpm) often have difficulty disassociating swallowing from breathing, thus increasing risk of aspiration with feedings.

Finally, premature infants, term infants and children are placed at greater risk for aspiration if they demonstrate any of the following characteristics:

- Difficulty coordinating respiration with swallowing
- Difficulty with state management
- Poor oral control

- Difficulties with any stage of swallowing (oral, pharyngeal or esophageal)
- Fatigue during the feeding
- Increased or decreased muscle tone
- Gastroesophageal reflux disorder
- Wheezing and Chronic cough
- Stridor
- Apnea
- Gagging and choking episodes

Aspiration and the Lungs

Infants and children aspirate small amounts when learning to swallow. However, if he or she aspirates large amounts of food or liquid or consistently aspirates smaller amounts, dangerous consequences can occur, specifically, to the lungs.

The overall health of an infant or child plays a significant role in placing the child at risk for aspiration. Chronic respiratory illness can cause aspiration, and constant aspiration can weaken the lungs and result in vulnerability to illnesses. Keep in mind that a patient may have been aspirating long before the development of pneumonia.

Premature infants who have a history of respiratory distress syndrome/hyaline membrane disease and/or bronchopulmonary dysplasia also suffer lung damage. The consequences of these illnesses make it difficult for the child to recover from an upper respiratory infection or pneumonia caused from aspiration.

Interestingly, Suzanne Evans Morris suggests that not all instances of aspiration affect the lungs in the same manner. Following are several features and variables of how aspiration can impact the lungs.

The *acidity* of the aspirated material has a major influence on the potential development of pneumonia. The higher the acid-level in the material, the greater the risk for pneumonia. Refluxed material places the patient at a greater risk for pneumonia, as compared to material that is more alkaline.

Foods or liquids that contain *fat molecules* (i.e. milk, yogurt, meat, and broth) are more dangerous to the lungs when aspirated than foods consisting primarily of water (i.e. fruits, vegetables and grains). Lungs and water are friendly; lungs and fat are not. On a daily basis, lungs handle and release water from the air we breathe. Fat, however, is a foreign substance and lungs have difficulty managing it.

Bacteria can influence the lungs. Bacteria are abundant in the oral cavity. It is important to develop an oral hygiene program for infants and children to reduce the amount of bacteria in the mouth especially if they have difficulty swallowing their secretions. Patients may be placed on medication to reduce the amount of saliva and to increase their ability to swallow their secretions. It should be noted however, that when saliva is thickened or reduced, the concentration of bacteria is increased within the remaining saliva. The patient is thus placed at risk for developing bacterial pneumonia if secretions are aspirated. If there is any question of aspiration, a thorough evaluation must be completed to avoid the potential harmful effect to the lungs.

Evaluation and Treatment of Pediatric Feeding Disorders: From NICU to Childhood

Signs and Symptoms of Aspiration

Behavioral observations can be telling in regards to the presence of aspiration. Do keep in mind, however, that some children show no visible signs of aspiration, yet are indeed aspirating. As part of your personal evaluation of the child, you may observe any combination of the following characteristics that may indicate aspiration is occurring. The child:

- Widens his or her eyes.
- Lifts his or her eyebrows.
- Exhibits a slight bluish color or color change around the eyes.
- Coughs or chokes during or after the feeding.
- Experiences bradycardia (heart rate drops below 100 bpm) during or after the feeding.
- Wheezes during or after the feeding.
- Gulps while swallowing.
- Exhibits a noisy, "wet" upper airway that can be heard during or after swallowing.
- May stop before the bottle/feeding is finished (child exhibits frequent incomplete feedings).
- Displays an aversion to feeding. He or she refuses to open his or her mouth to accept liquids and/or foods. Head turning, pushing away from the food or grimacing with acceptance of food are common symptoms.

In addition to the above on-site characteristics, the child may have

- A history of upper respiratory infection(s) and/or pneumonia. Pneumonia, however, may or may not be part of the child's history. Aspiration can result in formulation of scar tissue on the lungs without an immediate significant illness.
- A history of gastroesophageal or gastropharyngeal reflux.
- Significant weight loss.
- Oxygen saturation levels that register below 90.

Assessment of Aspiration

True documentation of aspiration during the pharyngeal phase of swallowing is determined by formal evaluations. The following methods are the current techniques most widely used:

- The <u>M</u>odified <u>B</u>arium <u>S</u>wallow studies (MBS) also known as
- The <u>V</u>ideofluroscopic <u>S</u>wallow <u>S</u>tudy (VFSS) and/or,
- The <u>F</u>iberoptic <u>E</u>ndoscopic <u>E</u>valuation of <u>S</u>wallowing (FEES).

Liquid and food of varying volumes and textures are administered by mouth. Swallowing efficiency and pharyngeal clearance is assessed.

Advocate for your patient during the studies. Make specific requests to insure a comprehensive study that addresses your patient's individual risk of aspiration with feedings is completed. Ask for specific food or liquid consistencies; indicate specific high risk swallowing time frames during the feeding (beginning, middle, end), as well as the positioning of the patient. Position the child as he is positioned by his caregiver for feedings and then make modifications and continue to assess position change and effect on the swallow during the study. The parent or primary caregiver should be present during the study and feed the child if at all possible. Use the child's own bottles, cups and utensils and interview the parent regarding liquids and foods that are challenging for the child to drink or eat at home. Document your requests and the findings in the event that aspiration may have been missed during the actual swallow study.

CERVICAL AUSCULTATION

Cervical auscultation (a subjective method of evaluating the swallow by placing a stethoscope at the right or left lateral portion of the neck and listening to the quality of the swallows) reveals premature spillage into the pharynx, delayed triggering of the swallow and or poor pharyngeal clearing.

Logemann describes the "clink" associated with the opening of the Eustachian tube and the "clunk" associated with the upper esophageal sphincter as the most reliable sounds during the swallow. The speech pathologist should first evaluate the sounds of respiration, define the inhalatory and exhalatory phase of the respiratory cycle, then determine if secretions are in the airway before or after the swallow, and note changes in secretion levels after the swallow.

Cervical auscultation can provide the therapist with information needed to recommend a complete swallow evaluation such as a modified barium swallow study or fiberoptic endoscopic evaluation of the swallow (FEES).

MODIFIED BARIUM SWALLOW STUDIES (MBS) OR VIDEOFLUROSCOPIC SWALLOW STUDIES (VFSS)

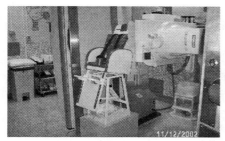
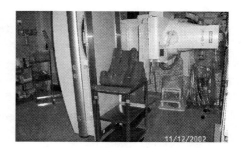

▲ *Mama Chair* ▲   ▲ *Tumbleform* ▲

The Mama Chair and Tumbleform seat are two types of equipment used to position infants and children in a natural feeding position during modified barium swallow studies. Obtaining a study mimicking a child's feeding position at home is important to determine the integrity of the swallow.

A modified barium swallow study yields a brief, momentary representation of the swallow. A speech pathologist and radiologist complete the study together. The study is meant to mimic an actual meal. The therapist adds contrast material (barium) to liquids and foods the child commonly consumes. The child is seated in a Tumbleform seat or the Mama Chair, which is similar to a high chair, but you can see through it during the study. The child is fed by the parent when possible using his own utensils and bottle/cup. The therapist and radiologist complete the study and then review it frame by frame to check again for trace aspiration.

Studies indicate that 50% of aspiration can be missed during modified barium swallow studies if they are not reviewed frame by frame by two observers. MBS is a relatively non-invasive assessment of the oral and pharyngeal stages of swallowing that uses barium as the swallowing content. Barium is visible via x-rays. MBS allows for the determination of consistencies and provides for safe swallowing conditions. Be sure to use a variety of consistencies of barium and slow-or high-flow nipples for a complete assessment of feeding capabilities.

Be aware that a patient can aspirate during a pause in the videofluoroscopy study. A MBS is only a "moment in time" and is not a guarantee that the child does not aspirate. The study needs to be repeated if feeding skills change as well as when the child grows, tone changes or if seizure activity increases. In some cases the most dangerous piece of information in a high risk child's medical history is a normal modified barium swallow study. Parents often feel that the child is completely safe because of the information shared during the assessment. Spend time educating parents about the limitations of this study and let them know that for children at risk, this is a test *series*, not a single event.

Both the MBS and/or VFSS studies allow the relatively non-invasive assessment of the oral and pharyngeal stage of swallowing and assist the therapist in determination of consistencies and conditions for safest possible swallowing.

FIBEROPTIC EVALUATION OF THE SWALLOW (FEES)

The fiberoptic endoscopic evaluation of swallowing, or FEES, is a diagnostic test that is used to identify patients who are at high risk for pulmonary aspiration. FEES is performed by passing a flexible scope into the oropharynx after anesthetizing the nares and nasopharynx.

A flexible fiberoptic laryngoscope is passed through the nasal cavity and placed in the pharynx at the level of the soft palate. Fiberoptic laryngoscopy is performed first and laryngeal biomechanics are evaluated. Particular attention is directed towards laryngeal inflammation, vocal fold mobility, glottic closure, and pharyngeal contraction. Pharyngeal anatomy and movement of pharyngeal and laryngeal structures can be evaluated during speech.

Management of secretions by FEES is completed by placing a small amount of green food coloring on the tongue. Accumulation of secretions in the valleculae or pyriform sinus or aspiration of secretions may be observed directly. This test is very helpful for evaluating children who may be aspirating saliva.

The examination then proceeds with the administration of several different food consistencies impregnated with methylene blue or food coloring. If several consistencies are tested, different colors are used so that they may be distinguished from each other on endoscopic evaluation. The test procedure generally begins with tastes of blue-colored applesauce. This food is one of the safest consistencies that can be tested and is usually well tolerated in terms of taste. A one-tablespoon bolus is placed on the tongue for adults; bolus size is individualized for children. The patient is asked to hold the food in his/her mouth and is then instructed to swallow. If the patient performs well (no evidence of deep penetration or aspiration), the applesauce is thinned with water to an intermediate (honey or nectar) consistency and the test is repeated. The applesauce is then thinned to a water consistency and the patient is given one tablespoon or appropriate size bolus for a child. If the patient does well he/she is challenged with the water consistency by taking several large sips using a straw. Bottle-feeding may also be observed. Many other consistencies of food, such as egg, toast, yogurt, cereal or hard foods such as carrots may be marked with food coloring and tested as indicated by the particular clinical needs of the patient. If the patient has a tracheotomy tube, the underside of the vocal cords can be viewed after the swallow to check for aspiration.

MBS VS. FEES: THE PROS AND CONS

- FEES can be used to assess sensation in the pharynx via a special scope that administers a calibrated puff of air onto the arytenoids or epiglottis. The ability to initiate airway closure with stimulation demonstrates airway protection.

- FEES and sensory testing may be valuable to evaluate swallowing safety in children who refuse to ingest adequate amounts of barium during MBS/VFSS.

- FEES can be used to evaluate aspiration of saliva.

- FEES does not provide information regarding the oral stage of swallowing but compares favorably with MBS for evaluation of the pharyngeal swallow. In several studies, when completed simultaneously, aspiration was missed using the MBS, but detected by FEES.

- FEES testing requires placement of a scope into the nasal cavity and many children may be frightened or distressed by this procedure. Numbing of the nasopharynx in some cases may also affect sensory feedback from pharynx. The procedure should be completed with care by a staff with experience working in pediatrics.

- FEES and a MBS can be completed simultaneously.

- According to Rudolph and Link, *"FEES is not a substitute for rigid endoscopy for evaluation of laryngeal anatomy. Laryngeal clefts may be overlooked during flexible endoscopy."*

Treatment of Aspiration

To aid in your treatment approach to aspiration, evaluate each stage of the swallow and determine what to do and how to promote safe, functional swallowing for that individual.

In addition to the MBS or FEES study, use cervical auscultation as a part of the assessment of the pharyngeal stage of the swallow. Cervical auscultation in no way replaces a MBS/FEES study. Remember, cervical auscultation does not give information on a child who aspirates silently.

Protecting the lungs is the main aspect of treatment. In fact, in some high-risk children, it is recommended that oral feeding be discontinued. Severe cases may warrant non-oral feedings. During this time, continue to apply oral sensory-motor techniques. The child, with the right care, may resume small, therapeutic oral feedings. Consider thermal stimulation (cold stimulus to the faucial arches or single cold bolus swallows) if the patient is an appropriate candidate.

The treatment methods you choose to use with a child who aspirates will be determined by the child's diagnosis and your clinical judgment of the events that lead to aspiration based on the results of the modified barium swallow study (MBS) or FEES and the feeding evaluation.

Remember, a g-tube or PEG tube is not the end of treatment of aspiration. Continue to work with these patients to help the child regain even limited oral feeding skills. Therapeutic tastes may consist of a few grains of pixie stix powder, but this can mean the world to parents!

REFERRAL OPTIONS

Everybody's a specialist—and isn't it fortunate we all have team members to turn to for help! A team approach to feeding management of a child with a history of aspiration is invaluable. If you do not have a feeding team to work with, pick up the phone and start making contacts. Network with other specialists and form a working relationship with occupational therapists, pediatric dietitians, nurses and physicians. Remember, they are looking for your help as well!

- Refer to a pediatric gastroenterologist if reflux and aspiration of gastric content is a concern.

- Refer to an ear, nose and throat specialist (ENT)/otolaryngologist for soft-tissue structural abnormalities or conditions that may increase the risk of aspiration.

- Confer with a medical team. Children who exhibit frank, silent aspiration and have a significant neurological history should be discussed with members of the medical team to create a comprehensive treatment program.

- Pediatric dietitians can provide vital information regarding the child's caloric needs and options for safely increasing calories of foods/liquids the child can consume.

- Positioning assistance is key to treatment of children who aspirate. Occupational and physical therapy co-treatment is strongly recommended.

PARENT EDUCATION

For parents of children who aspirate, parent education cannot be emphasized enough. A team approach to educating the family is strongly recommended. Explain aspiration in a way that parents understand the risk to their child's health if the current feeding patterns continue. The extended family and other caregivers should also be educated regarding aspiration for consistent care and to lend their support.

TREATMENT OPTIONS

Treatment includes making changes to the feeding procedures and ongoing re-assessment of the infant or child's feeding capabilities and factors that lead to aspiration.

Initially determine and monitor throughout treatment:

- The existing feeding technique(s)
- The fatigue level of the child
- The flow rate of the nipple
- The type of utensils used
- The feeding position, and
- The temperature and flavor of the foods as they impact bolus formulation and control

Depending on the patient, treatment options may include any or all of the following:

Thermal Stimulation

If the swallow is absent or delayed, and/or the gag and cough reflexes are absent or diminished, consider a trial of thermal stimulation techniques. Ideally, to be effective, thermal stimulation should be applied at least 5-6 times per day. Re-evaluate the child after the initial trial of thermal stimulation for any signs of an immediate change. Refer to Dr. Logemann's work on thermal stimulation for information regarding correct implementation of this treatment method.

Pediatric thermal stimulation can be applied in several manners. Apply ice-cold formula in single swallows via a pacifier or syringe. Use chilled pacifiers, or your iced gloved finger, Nuk Massage Brush, or ARK Probe to stimulate the faucial arches. Older children may allow the use of a chilled laryngeal mirror, followed by a light stroke down the larynx (externally) and a touch under the chin to encourage jaw closure. Use this technique carefully, so as not to create a negative experience. Wait to see if the child swallows. Re-assess the quality of the child's swallows daily or each session.

Drops of chilled formula via pacifier/syringe or Hazelbaker Finger Feeder for thermal stimulation and increased intra-oral awareness. Chilled bottle feedings may need to continue. Discuss with physician prior to initiating thermal stimulation, this technique may be contraindicated with some children.

External Pacing with Imposed Breaks

While bottle-feeding the well-positioned baby, tip the bottle down occasionally while leaving it inside the mouth. We tell parents we are briefly turning the nipple into a pacifier to avoid over-filling the mouth and also to allow an additional swallow to clear the pharynx. With older children, give them a "dry" swallow between bites or alternate consistencies of foods as needed.

Altering the Food Flow

Slower flow nipples or thickened feedings (consider risks of aspirating thickened formula first) may be used. Assess safety via modified barium swallow. Assess the consistencies of food given to older children. Do you need to alternate or manipulate the consistency of food to help the child have better control orally or clear the food better in the pharynx?

Altering Tastes and Temperatures

Strong food flavors and/or altered temperature can generate increased oral awareness and better control of the bolus in some children. This can occur because of the increased intensity of input to the sensory system. Remember the child may have a diminished sense of taste and very strong flavors (salsa, Tabasco sauce, A-1 sauce, a variety of different seasonings) may be used for feedings. Do not stay with baby food with older children. Purees don't have to be bland.

The Feeding Position

The desirable feeding position of the young infant is the semi-upright with *side tilt positioning* (similar to the position babies are in while breastfeeding). In this manner formula first collects in the buccal cavity and then enters the pharynx. Swaddling provides additional support to the body that provides stabilization for the oral structures to work optimally. With older infants with normal tone, only swaddling at the hips is necessary.

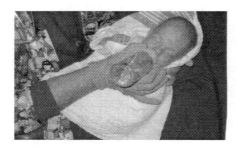

▲ Baby in side tilt ▲

Feeding a baby in a side tilt position (mimicking the position used for breastfeeding) allows the milk to collect in the cheek for a moment before it is swallowed. Amount of tilt of midline should be determined based on the individual infant's needs. This technique improves an infant's suck-swallow-breathe sequence.

The child should be in an upright position. Insure the child is well supported at the head, shoulder girdle, and pelvis and under the feet. Check the position of the head and neck carefully. Mimic the child's position yourself. If you feel increased laryngeal tension, make postural adjustments.

Prone positioning with an angle-neck bottle works for some infants (Pierre Robin Sequence, retracted tongue position). An older child may benefit from eating in a stander. Discuss appropriate posturing for your individual child with a physical or occupational therapist, if available.

Children with cerebral palsy may aspirate due to compensatory fixation patterns in the oral structures (abnormal tensions and posturing). Check the stability of their seating, if it provides ample support for appropriate feeding, and insure they have enough time to relax their body in the seating system prior to feeding. The child should be well positioned in the wheelchair 45-60 minutes prior to meals. Typically, children with cerebral palsy do not suddenly change their position. They require gradual postural changes. They receive feedback from their entire body while eating. For example, if the child is in cervical hyperextension so as to breathe more effectively, and quickly moves to a chin tuck, he may aspirate because he does not yet know how to swallow in the new position. Observe the child very carefully.

Oral-Motor Therapy

Oral motor therapy techniques can be used to meet the following goals:

- Strengthen the suck reflex,
- Improve oral transit time, and
- Improve bolus formulation and control.

Spoon Feeding

To reduce the size of the bolus (when spoon-feeding) or when working with children with poor oral control, allow the spoon to remain firmly on the lower lip/tongue for 5-10 seconds while the child takes in portions of the bolus and uses the spoon as a base of stability to prepare the bolus for swallowing. Jaw support, directly on the mandible, may also be needed.

Concentrated Feedings

Reduce intake demands by increasing the caloric intake (concentrate the feeding) to meet the nutritional needs of the infant or child. Formula is 20 kcal/oz and can be increased to 24 or 27 kcal/oz. This is most beneficial with children who aspirate at the end of feedings due to fatigue or have poor weight gain. Children whose nutritional status is poor are frequently quite weak. This weakness can impact feeding and place them at high-risk of aspiration.

Aspiration and Tracheotomy Tubes

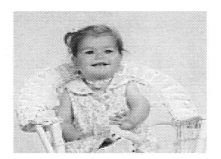

▲ Megan ▲

Prior to using a Passy Muir Valve, the blue dye that was added to Megan's feedings, was suctioned from her trach after each feeding detecting aspiration. While feeding with the valve on, the pressures for swallowing were normalized and there was no evidence of aspiration.

Research studies demonstrate that the use of a Passy-Muir Valve (PMV) in both neonates and pediatric patients significantly reduce episodes of aspiration. The literature on Passy Muir Valves states the following benefits for secretion management and swallowing:

- The PMV improves swallowing and reduces aspiration. It restores airflow and pressures in the throat that are needed to normalize the swallow. The design facilitates increased pharyngeal and laryngeal sensation and restores subglottic air pressures.

- The PMV helps decrease secretions by restoring airflow through the throat, nose and mouth. The airflow promotes evaporation of excess secretions. When wearing the PMV, a patient can close the vocal cords and build up enough pressure under the cords and within the lungs to produce a strong cough and clear secretions through the mouth.

- When the valve is placed, typically, a speech pathologist, respiratory therapist or pulmonary rehabilitation therapist present to assess the tolerance of the valve. The evaluation process includes the assessment of ease of inhalation and exhalation, pulse oximetry levels, vocal quality, and the child's comfort level and time tolerance of the valve.

- If the patient passes the evaluation process, a feeding trial may be initiated. Liquid or food is colored with blue food coloring to detect if ingested material is suctioned from the tracheotomy after the feeding.

The following sources provide additional information about the PMV:

The Laryngoscope, February 1996 Volume 10. Number 2 Part 1. Scintigraphic Quantification of Aspiration Reduction with the Passy-Muir Valve.

Annals of Otology, Rhinology, and Laryngology, April 1996, Volume 105 Number 4. Subglottic Air Pressure: A Key Component of Swallowing Efficiency.

Head and Neck, July/August 1995, Volume 17. Number 4. Effect of the Passy-Muir Valve on Aspiration in Patients with Tracheotomy.

CHAPTER THREE
▲
The Premature Infant: Evaluation and Treatment

"The preterm infant generates lower suction pressures that the term infant and may have difficulty adjusting to different nipple types."
--Rudolph and Link, 2002

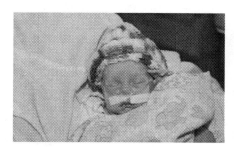

Advances in medical technology are resulting in infants surviving at earlier and earlier gestational ages. Medical and/or rehabilitation Professionals and school personnel will soon increase their caseloads with a new population of children who were born with extreme prematurity.

Practical Guidelines for Working with the Premature Infant

Assessment and treatment of premature infants is a challenge for the feeding professional. Following are some helpful, practical guidelines for working with premature infants in the medical setting.

THE ROLE OF THE SPEECH PATHOLOGIST

Typically, the speech pathologist assesses feeding skills, provides recommendations and communication to all staff for all shifts, educates the parents, and implements oral exercises with therapeutic feedings to improve oral sensory-motor capability and swallowing skills. The speech pathologist's primary role is *not to feed babies, but to make feeding therapeutic.* Most nurses are highly skilled feeders. The therapist manipulates the feeding to strengthen the oral musculature and develop appropriate activation of the oral musculature. Information gathered during daily therapy feedings is shared with nursing staff. To facilitate steady development, communicate each infant's feeding treatment program and progression to the nurses so the techniques can be implemented consistently.

Scheduling

NICU infants do not have adequate time for sleep, which is vital to their growth and development. Follow the infant's schedule for therapy visits and do not disturb them if you do not have a clear idea each day that you are in the unit of what your treatment program is and why you are there.

Continuous Education

It is vital that the speech pathologist in the NICU has a working knowledge of the medical issues and complications that can potentially impact the infant. Understanding of medical issues impacting each infant treated in the NICU is an absolute necessity for the therapist. Many disorders can have long-term effects on the baby's development. Respiratory problems, tone, joint stability and digestive tract disorders will continue to influence the child's feeding skills and overall development. Learn to implement a "whole body" treatment approach.

Continuous Improvement of Clinical Skills

Continuously work to advance your clinical skills. Learn from experienced therapists and the nurses in your unit. Meet with nurse educators and ask them for appropriate reading material to expand your knowledge base. Schedule time to observe the nurses feeding infants and let them teach you about preemies. Observe the disciplines of occupational and physical therapy for cross-training sessions.

Be Involved and Learn From Others

Discuss your recommendations with the physicians, respiratory therapists, nurses and parents, and work together as a team. In most cases, the nurses have worked with the infant for a long period of time. Nurses can provide valuable information to the therapist.

Communicate

Post treatment recommendations bedside. Make sure you communicate with all shifts so that all nurses are included in the treatment program. Place bright colored communication logs on the clipboard so the night nurses can write brief comments to the therapist regarding night feedings.

Be Sensitive to Family Needs

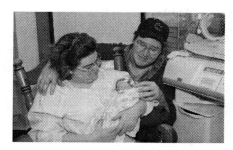

▲ Family of Three ▲

Education for changing diapers, giving baths, handling techniques, and feeding are provided so parents can take an active role in caring for their premature infant.

(Photo courtesy of St. John's Hospital, Springfield, Illinois.)

Be aware of and sensitive to the many stresses on the family from stays in the antenatal unit followed by the infant's hospitalization in the NICU. Bonding issues, financial stresses and fatigue may greatly impact the family and as a result, may impact the treatment.

Provide Parental Support

Teach the parents and include them in the treatment programs. Discuss and specify the care for the baby after discharge. Videotaped feeding instructions are a good idea to share with the parents, daycare providers, and appropriate others. Many infants' re-experience feeding problems with growth and changes occur in the oral cavity around 2 to 4 months of age. Increased saliva production can also be a problem for some NICU graduates. Advise the parents that they can contact you at any time after discharge if they start to experience difficulty with feedings.

Case Study: Jeremy, a NICU Infant

Let's begin our investigation of how to implement a thorough evaluation and implement specific treatment procedures with the premature infant with an example of an actual infant in the NICU. Please refer to Chapter 4 for a complete description of medical conditions common in premature infants.

HISTORY

Jeremy's medical history was significant. He was delivered at 24 weeks gestation, and had:
- Respiratory distress syndrome
- Bronchopulmonary dysplasia
- Necrotizing Enterocolitis
- Patent ductus arteriosis
- Grade III Intraventricular Hemorrhage
- Apnea
- Bradycardia
- Rickets, bone fractures and
- Liver damage from long-term TPN feedings

Interpretation of Medical History

Jeremy's medical history tells the therapist that he has a significant bleed in his brain and possible neurological issues as well as trouble breathing, which would most likely impact his coordination of the suck-swallow-breathe sequence. He had damage to his digestive tract and required surgery to remove diseased sections of his colon. He currently has symptoms of reflux and significant gastrointestinal discomfort after feeding. Jeremy will most likely require a special formula to meet his nutritional needs. Jeremy's heart condition is not that significant but his liver damage will affect his overall health, endurance and growth. Rickets and fractures indicate the need for special positioning techniques for feeding and daily care routine. Jeremy experienced many negative oral experiences to keep him alive and required long-term ventilation.

Social History

He has been in the hospital for a very long time and his mother is only 16-years-old. Jeremy's father is not involved in his life. Maternal grandmother will assist with Jeremy's care.

Evaluation

Assessment of Jeremy's oral peripheral mechanism revealed secretion management problems, very poor lip seal due to structural variation in the oral cavity, macroglossia, consistent open mouth posture, a very thin, inactive, upper lip and a high vaulted palate. Jeremy required supplemental oxygen that needed to be increased during feedings. The nurses reported long feedings with a pattern of choking and gagging at each feeding. Speech therapy was consulted to evaluate and to assist the nursing staff with feedings and also to provide parent education regarding special feeding techniques.

EVALUATION FINDINGS

Jeremy was a very sick infant with a strong desire to nipple. His oral reflexes were intact and he eagerly turned toward the pacifier as non-nutritive sucking was assessed. A strong tongue thrust pattern and intermittent tremor were noted and Jeremy could not seal his mouth around the nipple. He was constantly spilling liquid from his mouth and ingesting large quantities of air with his feedings. He had been vomiting after feeding attempts. Past feedings were discussed with the nurses who knew him well. They reported very long, difficult feedings. They also expressed concerns that Jeremy was aspirating while nippling.

He was briefly evaluated by the speech therapist on the Ross hospital-brand yellow standard nipple used to feed infants in the unit and Jeremy presented with severe oral spillage, gagging, poor-to-absent bolus control, watery eyes, desaturation while feeding and gulpy swallows. Cervical auscultation revealed multiple swallows were needed to clear the pharynx.

The swallow was very inefficient because Jeremy could not build up negative pressure within the oral cavity due to his inability to seal his lips around the nipple.

TREATMENT PLAN

The speech therapist chose a market brand nipple, the Parent's Choice 0+ silicone nipple from Luv-n-Care because of the slow flow rate and the large diameter of the nipple. This nipple is too large in diameter for many NICU babies; however, due to Jeremy's variation of oral structures this was an appropriate choice. The firmness of this nipple would still provide the much-needed input to the midline tongue to encourage tongue grooving and assist lip seal, which would improve bolus control.

Side-tilt positioning was attempted to compensate for poor-to-absent bolus formulation, so milk would collect in the lateral sulci (cheeks) prior to entering the pharynx. External pacing was provided by tipping the bottle down to stop the flow of milk to allow an additional swallow while leaving the nipple in the mouth to maintain organized state. Firm proprioceptive input was provided to the body via a pillow due to the concerns regarding rickets and bone fractures. Cheek and jaw support was provided with a rolled burp cloth under the chin with support to the cheek tissue with the speech therapist's hands. Jeremy nippled 30 cc's for the therapist without desaturation. As the flow rate was decreased using the Parent's Choice nipple, he was able to suck with increased activation of the oral musculature.

An oral exercise program was developed to improve strength and movement of the lips, cheeks and tongue. The therapist used the Soothie pacifier to provide deep input to the midline tongue to improve tongue cupping. Jeremy's feedings were closely monitored. He fed well with the Parent's Choice nipple over a 24-hour trial period; however, gulpy swallows were reported at the end of feedings. Nippling was limited to 20 minutes maximum with a three-minute rest period mid-feeding. The remainder of the feeding was given via the nasogastric tube. The therapist took the time to explain to physicians, nurses and family members that feedings in the beginning of the treatment program were simply for "practice" and they were cautioned that intake amount would be very limited.

Progress would be measured at this phase of treatment based on activating and strengthening the oral musculature, not by caloric intake. The first in a series of modified barium swallow studies was completed to rule out silent aspiration. Jeremy was at risk for aspiration but with appropriate positioning and flow rate of the Parent's Choice nipple he safely consumed 40 cc's. Parent education sessions began and Jeremy's mother and grandmother were trained with verbal, hand over hand, written instructions with photographs to assist with education. Recommendations were posted for all shifts of the nursing staff so feeding technique would remain consistent feeder to feeder. Consultation with occupational therapy was recommended by the speech therapist, but evaluation was not ordered by the physician.

RESULTS

As strength of Jeremy's oral musculature increased and bolus formulation skills improved, he was later placed on the 6+ Parent's Choice nipple, which has a faster flow rate. He needed this increased flow rate due to fatigue with feeding, however, until he had a foundation of appropriate feeding skills, increasing the rate of the feeding too early in the treatment program would have placed him at a very high risk for aspiration. Jeremy received the majority of his nutrition via a silastic feeding tube until he was able to nipple full feedings. This gave the speech therapist adequate time to improve his feeding skills. Changing Jeremy to a slow flow nipple at the beginning of his treatment program gave him the chance to develop the skills and strengthen the musculature for more efficient sucking. A change from the Parent's Choice 0+ to the 6+ therefore, was easy for him as the nipples were identical except for flow rate.

Jeremy was slowly weaned from supplemental oxygen and began taking more each feeding. A four-hour schedule was attempted and with longer rest periods between feedings, Jeremy began to nipple well. Feedings were concentrated to 24-k/cal, which reduced intake demands.

Parent education sessions were repeated and the family was urged to continue therapy recommendations. The family was provided a supply of nipples when Jeremy left the NICU to go home. Because this product is distributed by department stores such as Wal-Mart, the family would have no problems finding replacements as needed.

Jeremy was referred to the outpatient feeding team clinic for a recheck two weeks after discharge. As Jeremy was at high risk for acquiring additional feeding and developmental problems in the future, he began an outpatient treatment program with speech therapy and occupational therapy. Weekly weight checks continued and were reported to the feeding team.

Evaluation and Treatment

Do your homework! Investigate the infants' complete medical history by reviewing the chart (or other appropriate file) and talking to nurses, parents, and other caregivers. Get their impressions and descriptions of the feeding problem. Check daily-notes from nursing staff. Make a note of the infant's food intake over the previous 36-48 hours. Note patterns of alertness and intake.

ASSESSING STATE LEVEL

State management refers to how a baby responds to sights, sounds, and movement in his environment, as well as handling. Assess state while the baby is resting in the isolette and continue to assess changes during cares, handling, initiation of feeding, nippling and after the feeding has been completed. According to Brazelton and Als there are six levels of state. They include:

The Premature Infant: Evaluation and Treatment

1. *Deep Sleep:* An infant in deep sleep is characterized by:
   - Momentary regular breathing
   - Closed eyes
   - No eye movements under closed lids
   - Relaxed facial expression
   - No spontaneous activity
   - Isolated startles
   - Jerky movements or tremors, and
   - Other behavior characteristics of light sleep state

2. *Light Sleep:* An infant in light sleep emits the impression of a "noisy" state. Light sleep is characterized by:
   - Closed eyes
   - Rapid eye movements can be observed under closed lids
   - Low activity level with diffuse or disorganized movements
   - Respirations that are irregular
   - Numerous sucking and mouthing movements
   - Numerous whimpers
   - Numerous facial twitches
   - Much facial grimacing
   - An isolated sigh or smile

3. *Drowsy or Semi-Dozing:* An infant that is drowsy or semi-dozing is characterized by:
   - Either open or closed eyes
   - Eyelids that flutter or blink in an exaggerated manner
   - A glassy veiled look, if eyes are open
   - A variable activity level that may or may not be interspersed mild startles from time to time
   - Diffused movement
   - Fussing and/or
   - Numerous vocalizations, whimpers, and facial grimacing

4. *Alert:* An infant that is alert exhibits the following characteristics:
   - Clearly awake, quiet, and reactive, but has his eyes open intermittently.
   - Emits minimal motor activity
   - Eyes are half open, with a glazed or dull look; gives the impression of little involvement
   - Focused, yet seems to look through, rather than at, an object or the examiner

5. *Active:* An infant that is active exhibits the following characteristics:
   - Eyes may or may not be open, but infant is clearly awake and aroused
   - Indicates appropriate motor arousal
   - Has appropriate muscle tonus

33

- Is mildly distressed as exhibited by appropriate facial expression, grimacing, or other signs of discomfort
- Fussing is diffuse

6. *Crying:* A crying infant exhibits the following characteristics:
   - Intense crying as indicated by intense grimacing and "cry face"
   - The cry sound may be strained or weak or even absent
   - May see rhythmic, intense crying which is robust, vigorous and strong in sound

It is vital to look not only at the infant's current state, but also the range of the infant's state, the frequency with which they change state, how smoothly they transition between states, and what physiological effects are elicited in attempts to maintain a specific state.

Appetite is also affected by emotional state; infants who are not nurtured reduce their food intake. Infants with subtle feeding disorders are less resilient in responding to difficult environments and emotional deprivation than normal infants.

ASSESSING ORAL REFLEXES

When an infant is born, he or she is born with several reflexes. They include rooting, sucking, swallowing, the phasic bite, the transverse tongue, gagging, and coughing. Prior to assessing these reflexes, do determine if the infant can tolerate touch to the oral musculature.

The Root Reflex

Begin with assessing the root reflex. Stroke down the center of the lower lip; watch for the mouth to open in response to the stimulus. Repeatedly stimulate the root reflex if it appears to be absent.

In therapy, spend time working on this reflex. A root often results in appropriate downward position of the tongue, spontaneous opening of the mouth and improved organization and readiness for introduction of the nipple into the mouth.

The Sucking Reflex

Next, assess the non-nutritive suck. Place your finger on top of the baby's tongue. The tongue should go down and cup around your finger. You should feel the pull of negative pressure when you remove your finger.

The Swallowing Reflex

Note the following during swallowing: Are the cheeks active? Is there a sucking pattern or a munching pattern? Is the jaw stable? Does the baby demonstrate a suck that can potentially propel liquid posteriorly for an efficient swallow?

In addition, observe how the baby handles the breathing and sucking sequence. Did the baby desaturate? Did you observe any head bobbing from increased respiratory effort? From this investigation, begin to determine if single bolus swallows is the level of treatment, or bottle use? This is the stage of the assessment to determine if it is safe to attempt bottle use, or not.

The Phasic Bite

Assess the phasic bite by rubbing the molar area left and right. You should feel a firm bite on both sides of equal pressure. A very strong clamping-type bite indicates a tonic bite reflex and is not normal.

The Transverse Tongue Reflex

Rub the sides of the tongue to assess transverse tongue movement. The tongue should move laterally with stimulation. Is there equal and adequate movement?

The Gag Reflex

The gag reflex is a protective reaction that triggers in response to touching the posterior region of the tongue. When assessing the gag, with posterior palpation, the gag should trigger easily. An absent gag reflex raises a developmental red flag. The absent gag can be indicative of the need for a thorough neurological consultation.

The Cough Reflex

If you do not directly observe the cough reflex during your assessment, check with others (the nurse/staff) regarding their observations. The cough is important. It is the protective reflex for liquid intake. Premature infants may have very diminished respiratory function and their cough may be weak and ineffective.

ASSESSING NUTRITIVE SUCKING/SWALLOWING

The nutritive suck should look "coordinated". Ideally, the baby has a calm look on his or her face and should demonstrate sucking bursts and pauses of equal duration. Swallows should not be audible. Closely observe breathing pattern, color, heart rate, state, and comfort level. Can the baby maintain ventilation? Do pauses help? How long did the baby take to finish the feeding?

Does the infant demonstrate signs of GI distress during the feeding? Were there changes mid-feed or toward the end of the feeding that put the baby at risk? How strong is the swallow?

What are the nurse's complaints? Are there more problems during the night or the day?

Watch for and analyze patterns, and use cervical auscultation to assist in the evaluation of the swallow during the feeding.

ASSESSING INFANT CUES

Following are physical cues that an infant may demonstrate indicating signs of readiness to approach him or her, as well as indicators of coping behaviors and distress cues. These cues can be helpful in not only reading the signals to approach or not approach an infant, but also the reliability of your evaluation results.

Approach-Readiness Cues
- Smiling
- Cooing
- Little active movement
- Alertness
- Relaxed face
- "O" face

Coping Cues
- Hands to face, mouth or midline
- Flexor posturing
- Grasp
- Fisting
- Sucking
- Change in state (lower level)

Stress Signs
- Burping
- Spitting up
- Arching/posturing of trunk or extremities
- Changes in vital signs
- Changes in color
- Hiccups
- Irritability
- Yawning
- Squirming or increased activity level

FACILITATING A CALM STATE AND STABILITY

Identifying an infant's medical condition, tone, and individual sensitivities and responses will facilitate the selection of the most effective techniques to help manage an infant in distress. Consulting an occupational therapist is recommended.

Provision of developmentally supportive positioning interventions may promote a calm state and physiological stability for the high-risk infant. For example, if the infant is motorically stressed, help him reorganize by
- Holding his extremities in flexion close to his body until calm, thereby decreasing unnecessary energy expenditure and encouraging self-regulation.
- Swaddling

The Premature Infant: Evaluation and Treatment

- Facilitating non-nutritive sucking, or
- Providing rhythmical vestibular input to help soothe and reorganize the infant.

In addition, provide momentary time-out from incoming stimuli when a baby is stressed and disorganized to allow him to draw fully on self-regulatory abilities.

Observe the baby for avoidance behaviors (gaze aversion, regurgitation, crying, increased extension patterns) in response to movement transitions or particular positions. When repositioning an infant, contain the limbs to help the infant maintain stability and stay in control; use slow, gentle movements.

MONITORING HEART AND RESPIRATORY RATES

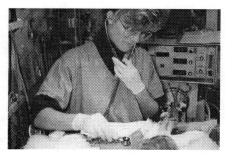

Respiratory therapists are an important part of the treatment team in the NICU.

(Photo courtesy of St. John's Hospital, Springfield, Illinois.)

▲ *Respiratory Therapist listening to a child with stethoscope* ▲

Check with the nurse to determine what is the "normal" heart rate of the infant. A premature infant's heart rate should be between 160-180 bpm with an increase of 10bpm with the exertion of feeding. Respiratory rate should remain between 30-60 breaths per minute. A heart rate of 100 or below is called bradycardia and a heart rate that exceeds 180 is called tachycardia.

HANDLING AND POSITIONING THE INFANT

In the premature infant, do keep in mind that the vestibular, visual and auditory systems are not fully developed. Keep the lights low, sound to a minimum and move the baby slowly. Do not rock or talk to the baby while feeding.

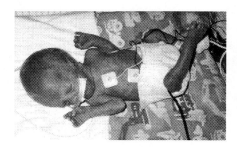

◄ *Because a premature baby lacks strength and stability in their joints, gravity draws the infant into a surface. The need for developmental positioning is critical.*

Evaluation and Treatment of Pediatric Feeding Disorders: From NICU to Childhood

The baby should be swaddled firmly up to and around the shoulders, hands should be up by the face and the blanket should be loosened around the chest so as not to restrict breathing. Also check that the diaper is not too tight around the waist so as to restrict breathing.

Positioning is crucial to develop effective feeding. Keep in mind that physiological flexion supports feeding. The baby needs to maintain the airway, regulate his breathing and swallow safely while maintaining an organized state.

Position of the head, neck, and shoulder girdle should be closely monitored. The baby can be fed en face, in modified sidelying or semi-upright. Assess which position maintains head and trunk alignment and seems to work for the baby. We recommend semi-upright in modified sidelying position, similar to the position a breastfeeding baby. This position allows the milk to enter the buccal area first, before moving into the pharynx. This provides the infant improved control of the liquid bolus. Supine positioning can lead to incorrect head and neck alignment as well as an increased risk of positional otitis media and aspiration. (Lawrence)

When is Baby Ready for Nippling?

Age, although not the only factor, is the basic criteria for nippling-readiness. The baby should be at least 34 weeks post-conceptional age. An infant less than 34 weeks does not have the skills to swallow with control and is too young to support and stabilize the airway. Strength, motility and coordination of pharyngeal muscles used for swallowing correlates with the 34-week developmental progression. Many infants are not ready to nipple until they reach 37 weeks gestation.

In premature infants, mouthing patterns that emerge as early as 13 weeks gestation, persist until approximately 32 weeks gestation. "At 32 weeks, a disorganized pattern of sucking bursts and pauses are observed, being replaced by a stable pattern of rhythmical sucking and swallowing at 34 to 36 weeks gestation." (Rudolph)

Evaluate the infant overall, in regard to state, endurance, weight and condition. Nippling-readiness is frequently misjudged by non-nutritive sucking on a pacifier. Non-nutritive and nutritive sucking are two different acts and cannot be equated to readiness for oral intake.

The preterm infant generates lower suction pressures than the term infant and may have difficulty adjusting to different nipple types. (Rudolph and Link) Nipple selection must match the infant's needs and should be used consistently by all of those involved in feeding the child.

The head, neck and shoulder girdle support the trachea and larynx. Assess the infant's motor control or refer or co-treat with occupational therapist or physical therapist to analyze the infant's motor skills.

Another critical issue is respiratory status. If increased respiratory rate and/or heart rate, retractions and excessive use of accessory muscles of the rib cage are noted during non-nutritive sucking, carefully consider delaying nippling. Take into account the extreme risks of nippling a baby with these symptoms.

Disorganized breathing can easily disrupt the swallow. Feeding is coordination of the suck, swallow, breathe sequence and is the hardest work the infant has to do each day. You may recommend oral stimulation, therapeutic tastes and co-treatment with OT and/or PT to lay the capability foundation to move to nippling.

To be ready to attempt nippling, the baby should be able to maintain a quiet alert state for at least ten minutes.

NICU nurses and staff are under pressure to get infants nippling as soon as possible. Be an advocate for the infant and promote understanding of the physiological reasons why nippling too early can cause additional problems and possibly lengthen the hospital stay. Typically, therapy cannot change the neurodevelopmental level of the baby or the baby's readiness for nippling. However, if the physician orders the baby to receive PO feeds, the speech therapist can help to make the baby as safe as possible.

Feeding therapy can also break-up, modify and in some cases prevent abnormal feeding patterns from developing.

Nipple Choice

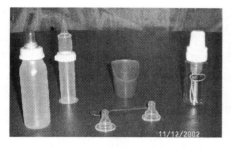

These feeding devices are just a few of the tools used to help build strength and stability in the oral musculature while feeding. When choosing an appropriate tool for feeding you must know the impact to the oral, pharyngeal, and esophageal stages of the swallow.

▲ *Bottles, Nipples, Spoons* ▲

High-flow nipples are designed to reduce the feeding effort for premature infants. However, they transfer the work from the oral stage to the pharyngeal stage due to the increased flow rate.

Pink, blue, red and Nuk brand nipples are often used in the NICU with infants who have a weak suck. If the tongue is too weak to suck, the tongue is too weak to propel the liquid back for swallowing. Hypercarbia, acidosis and apnea and bradycardia can occur.

The yellow nipple is generally recommended for feeding premature infants. The role of the speech pathologist is to educate physicians, staff, and families of the risks in using high flow nipples.

RISKS OF HIGH-FLOW-RATE NIPPLES

Current research (Lan et al 1997) suggests that reduced flow rate produces a more active suck and that premature infants take more per feeding over a 24-hour period with a slow to medium-flow nipple. This study evaluated infants on the Ross standard yellow nipple and the Ross red preemie nipple for comparison. Using the yellow standard medium flow Ross nipple, infants had greater intake over the course of the 24-hour period and were able to maintain improved ventilation during feeding.

When the flow-rate of the nipple is too high, the following consequences may occur:

- Loss of bolus control
- Fluid spills toward the airway and can splash over into the pharynx
- Inadequate time to breathe with decreased ventilation
- Increased risk of microaspiration
- Fatigues the infant due to greatly increased work of feeding
- Increased risk of reflux
- Impairs infant's ability to maintain state/coordination
- Risk of developing aversion to feeding

Please refer to the nipple comparison information in Chapter 11 for details regarding nipple choice after discharge from the NICU.

Fostering Parent-Education

Parent education is extremely important. Parents feel many conflicting emotions during their infant's stay in the NICU. Education, support and encouragement from medical staff are extremely beneficial. Helping a parent understand their infant's level of communication via the infant's behavior can help them respond to and interact with their baby successfully.

Staff can support this interaction by teaching parent's to recognize stress signs, use consoling measures, and provide care-giving responsibilities. Specific interactive activities can be demonstrated for the parent. Recorded tapes of the parent's voices can be played periodically when they are not present with their child. These activities help parents bond with their baby.

Let parents voice their concerns and expectations for their child. Discuss discrepancies between expectations and reality through team meetings with the family. The physician, social worker and nursing staff can direct these interactions.

Provide information to the family regarding therapy sessions. Contact them when they are absent. Train the parent to reassess feeding behaviors daily. Give them detailed instructions regarding their infant's positioning needs and specific feeding strategies.

CHAPTER FOUR
▲
The Premature Infant: Medical Reference Guide

"In the preterm infant, the coordination of sucking, swallowing and breathing is not fully mature. Preterm infants tend to hold their breath for several seconds, during which time a number of sucks and swallows occur. This pattern of multiple swallows without respiration decreases with increasing postconceptual age."
--Hanlon MB, et al, 1997

At this point in time, premature infants are surviving deliveries as early as 21-22 weeks gestation. Due to their early birth, they have conditions that can impact their growth and development in a variety of ways. Medical information can be vast and overwhelming, but the child's history is extremely important to the feeding therapist. Prematurity does not really end, premature infants carry their history with them. These children have significant differences in joint stability, tone and strength, as well as neurological, respiratory and digestive system problems that can impact successful oral feeding.

It is also important to understand the experiences of the mother during pregnancy and delivery of such a fragile child. The therapist needs to look closely at the child's medical history to truly know the patient and develop an understanding of the long-term effects of his prematurity.

Prematurity and the Risk Factors

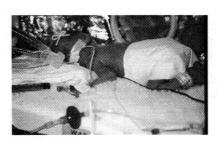

The following is a detailed and extensive reference, written to assist the therapist in understanding the complexities of prematurity and their patient's medical history. (Beachy and Deacon, 1993) Also discussed, are the long-term outcomes that may be observed when working with NICU graduates.

The normal length of pregnancy is 280 days or 40 post-menstrual weeks. The first trimester is 0 to 12 weeks, the second trimester is 13 to 27 weeks and the third trimester is 28 to 40 weeks.

Pre-term delivery is less than 37 weeks, term delivery is 38 to 42 weeks, and post-term delivery is more than 42 weeks.

Abortion is defined as terminated pregnancy prior to 24 weeks and includes spontaneous and elective abortions as well as ectopic pregnancies. Multiparas (multiple births) may have a higher rate of complications.

Basic to the investigating the mother's history, use the acronym "GPAL" as a key association to glean the following information:

- G is gravidity (number of pregnancies),
- P is parity (number of births),
- A is number of abortions, and
- L is number of live births

There are several maternal factors that can influence prematurity of birth. Following is a list of the most frequent causes and contributing factors:

- Poor prenatal care
- Poor nutrition
- Low socioeconomic status
- Recurrent abortion
- Substance abuse
- Maternal fever
- Prolonged rupture of the membranes
- Chorioamnionitis
- Urinary tract infection
- Prolonged, difficult labor, and premature labor
- History of infection (hepatitis, HIV, STD's)
- Smoking
- Substance abuse
- Emotional problems, and a
- Significant genetic history

Antenatal Steroid Therapies for the Mother

BETAMETHAZONE

Betamethazone is a two to three day course of steroids administered to the mother prior to delivery to help mature the infant's lungs. If labor cannot be stopped the infant is given Survanta, a steroid to help replace the detergent-like substance surfactant that is produced by type II pneumocytes around 28 weeks gestational age. Surfactant makes the lungs more elastic and less prone to collapse or atelactisis.

MAGNESIUM SULFATE THERAPY

Magnesium Sulfate therapy is used to stop labor and can be given as a CNS depressant to prevent convulsions. It has a smooth-muscle relaxant effect and reduces the mother's blood pressure. Magnesium crosses the placenta and affects the baby. Muscle relaxant may cause the baby to experience increased respiratory distress and may also affect the gut and give the baby an ileus. An ileus is an area of inactive gut and is characterized by severe colicky pain, dehydration and obstruction may also occur. The baby will be assessed for signs of hypermagnesemia including:

- Weakness and lethargy
- hypotonia
- flaccidity
- respiratory depression
- poor suck
- decreased GI motility,
- hypotension
- urinary retention, and
- increase in atrioventricular and ventricular conduction when high levels of magnesium sulfate are given near the time of delivery. The body excretes magnesium sulfate over the course of a few days.

The baby is kept NPO until the levels are lower. There is controversy over the NPO status that exists in some NICU's; some physicians will allow feedings if baby seems stable. During NPO status the baby is generally fed by TPN (total parenteral nutrition). It is felt that the baby does not actively experience hunger until the suck reflex emerges at approximately 34 weeks.

Complications of Pregnancy and Delivery
(Beachy and Deacon, 1993)

The following potential complications are listed alphabetically for easy identification.

ABRUPTIO PRACENTAE

Definition

Abruptio placentae is defined as sudden and premature separation of the placenta from the uterine wall during pregnancy or labor. It occurs in one in 100 to 250 deliveries.

Symptoms

Abruptio placentae is characterized by sharp, continuous abdominal pain, a board-like and tender abdomen, dark or bright red vaginal bleeding (ranging from spotting to frank hemorrhage; the blood may be concealed behind the placenta), wine colored amniotic fluid, and enlargement of the uterus due to blood accumulation.

Treatment

Bedrest may help if bleeding is not severe. C-section delivery is completed if the bleeding is severe.

Complications

There can be maternal complications. They include: anemia, hypovolemic shock, DIC, kidney necrosis and renal shutdown, and death. The fetus can exhibit weak or absent heart tones, tachycardia and late decelerations. Fetal complications may include neonatal anemia, hypoxia, asphyxia and death.

ANTEPARTUM CONDITIONS

Definition

Pregnancy-Induced Hypertension (PIH), which includes pre-eclampsia and eclampsia, is a major cause of perinatal morbidity and mortality in the United States. It is also the third leading cause of maternal death in this country. Pathophysiologic events in PIH are vasospasm, hematologic changes, deposition of fibrin and fibrinogen in vessels, hypovolemia secondary to fluid shifts and increased CNS irritability.

Etiology

The exact cause of PIH has not been determined.

Symptoms

The mother presents with increased blood pressure (140/90 or above, or a rise of 30 mm Hg/systolic or 15 mm Hg/diastolic or more over the early pregnancy baseline) after the twentieth week of the pregnancy. Other signs include elevated protein in the urine due to decreased renal perfusion, edema due to sodium retention and decreased plasma colloid osmotic pressure, headache, hyper-reflexia with clonus, visual and retinal changes, irritability, nausea and vomiting, epigastric pain, dyspnea and oliguria.

Complications

Complications for the mother include: Eclampsia (grand mal seizure), cardiopulmonary failure, peripartum cardiomyopathy, hepatic rupture, cerebrovascular accident, renal cortical necrosis, disseminated intravascular coagulation (DIC), HELLP syndrome and retinal detachment.

Complications for the baby include: Premature placental aging, placental infarction and decreased amniotic fluid, abruptio placentae, IUGR (intrauterine growth retardation) secondary to decreased placental blood flow, fetal distress and preterm delivery.

The Premature Infant: Medical Reference Guide

Treatment

Treatment of pre-eclampsia includes hospitalization with complete bed-rest in left lateral recumbent position, limited stimulation (visitors and noise), seizure precautions, frequent assessment of all systems, high-protein and moderate sodium diet, blood work, placental-fetal function tests and medications. Fetal monitoring should be completed to check for hypoxia from the sudden decrease in maternal blood pressure.

Treatment for eclampsia includes care of the mother during the convulsion, support breathing management, oxygen, suctioning, fetal monitoring, magnesium sulfate IV push, Apresoline (for antihypertensive effect) and delivery by induction or cesarean when the woman and fetus recover. The newborn baby should be assessed for IUGR, hypoxia and acidosis.

APNEA OF PREMATURITY

Definition

Apnea is cessation of breathing for 15 to 20 seconds or more. It is associated with color change (pale, purple or blue) and is associated with bradycardia (low heart rate). Apnea of prematurity is due to immature respiratory centers in the brain. Premature infants normally have bursts of full breaths followed by shallow ones or pauses. Apnea is more common during sleep. All apnea is not due to prematurity.

Etiology

Apnea can be caused by: Infection, low blood sugar, PDA, seizure, high or low body temperature, brain injury, insufficient oxygen or obstruction in the airway.

Treatment

Treatment consists of medications that stimulate breathing, such as aminophylline and theophylline, CPAP, periodic stimulation and mechanical ventilation, if severe.

BRONCHOPULMONARY DYSPLASIA (BPD)

Definition

Bronchopulmonary dysplasia (BPD) is a progressive lung disease seen in infants who have received high concentrations of oxygen during mechanical ventilation.

45

Symptoms

In addition to having a more difficult time growing, the child with BPD exhibits rapid or difficult breathing, wheezing, and wet, crackling sound to lungs, heard via auscultation. The infant may have complications of intermittent bronchospasms, recurrent infections, upper respiratory infections, pneumonia, otitis media and congestive heart failure.

Treatment

Infants are treated by continued respiratory support, oxygen after extubation to avoid hypoxia and the use of diuretics to control fluid retention leading to pulmonary edema that is frequently seen with BPD. Steroids are given as needed. Bronchodialators are given to reduce airway resistance and to control wheezing. Optimal nutritional support, and respiratory therapy is needed to compensate for increased work of breathing and fluid restriction. Infant may require a tracheotomy tube and long-term vent support.

Complications

Fluid restriction may reduce pulmonary edema and right sided heart failure. A cardiac evaluation is usually completed to investigate for complications. BPD can be a fatal complication. The incidence is decreasing with the increase of advanced technology in mechanical ventilation. Because new lung tissue grows between the ages of one year and three years, prognosis may improve over time. Many children with BPD have significant feeding problems.

CONGENITAL DIAPHRAGMATIC HERNIA

Definition

The diaphragm is a broad muscle that is involved in respiration of the lungs by contracting and relaxing. The diaphragm forms at 8 weeks gestation. This occurs by the merging of two membranes to close off the open area between the chest and abdomen. If it does not close completely, a defect, called diaphragmatic hernia is created. Hernia refers to both the hole in the diaphragm muscle and the protrusion of the abdominal organs into the chest. The stomach, small and large bowel and other organs such as the kidney and liver can herniate.

Complications

Complications result as the lung on the affected side and the opposite side cannot grow to full capacity. Shortly after delivery, the infant swallows air while crying and the bowel in the chest inflates with air and further compromises the insufficient lung.

Treatment

Children with severe lung deficiency may be placed on ECMO to allow circulation of the blood through an external oxygenator pump. Surgery is required.

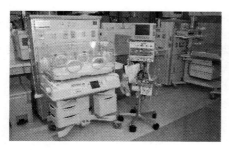

▲ *Isolette with a conventional ventilator* ▲

A preterm infant will spend much time in an isolette continuing his development in this "womb-like" environment. A conventional ventilator breathes for the baby completely and allows the physician and respiratory therapist to determine the number of breaths per minute and the depths of the breaths.

(Photo courtesy of St. John's Hospital, Springfield, Illinois.)

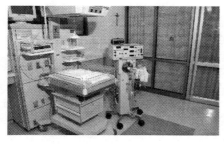

▲ *Warming bed with ossocilating ventilator* ▲

An ossocilating ventilator keeps the lungs inflated by providing continuous puffs of air (approximately 300 puffs per minute) and allows the infant to breath on his own.

(Photo courtesy of St. John's Hospital, Springfield, Illinois.)

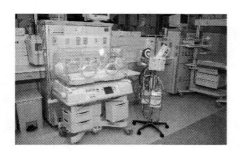

▲ *Isolette with CPAP* ▲

CPAP provides continuous positive pressure to maintain the tiniest of air sacs in the lungs from collapsing.

(Photo courtesy of St. John's Hospital, Springfield, Illinois.)

DISSEMINATED INTRAVASCULAR COAGULATION (DIC)

Definition

DIC is an acquired hemorrhagic disorder associated with underlying disease. It is manifested as an uncontrolled activation of coagulation and fibrinolysis. Consumption of clotting factors is initiated by the release of thromboplastic material from damaged or diseased tissue into circulation. It is characterized by generalized, multiple site bleeding.

Precipitating Factors

Precipitating factors can include: pre-eclampsia, placental abnormalities, fetal distress with hypoxia and acidosis, dead twin fetus, traumatic delivery, infection, severe Rh incompatibility and thrombocytopenia.

Complications

Complications include organ failure secondary to ischemia and necrosis (especially renal) and intraventricular hemorrhage.

HELLP SYNDROME

Definition

Hellp syndrome is a unique variant of pre-eclampsia (toxemia). It has the following characteristics: H (hemolysis, breaking down of the red blood cells), EL (elevated liver enzymes), and LP (low platelet count).

Complications

The majority of babies born to mothers with HELLP syndrome do very well. However, it can be fatal to both mother and baby, and can occur in tandem with pre-eclampsia (high blood pressure, protein in the urine and swelling). If baby is less than 1000 grams, he or she have may have a longer hospital stay and an increased chance of requiring mechanical ventilation. There is also an increased mortality rate for LBW infants. Most infant deaths are a result of abruption of the placenta, intrauterine asphyxia and extreme prematurity.

Treatment

The only definitive treatment for HELLP syndrome is delivery of the infant.

HEMATOCRIT LEVEL

Hematocrit (HCT) is the volume or percentage of red blood cells (RBC) in the circulating blood. A normal newborn infant HCT level is 44% to 72%. Hemoglobin is a component of RBC's and is used to determine anemia. Normal newborn HGB is 14.5 to 22.5g/dl. The RBC's and HGB will fall in the first month of life averaging 11 to 17 g/dl for HGB.

If HCT is too low, anemia occurs. The infant is pale and weak. If HCT is too high, it can indicate polycythemia, which causes thick, sludgy blood. The baby will have a red, ruddy color. The thick blood does not deliver oxygen to the tissues therefore an exchange transfusion is completed to dilute the blood and provide better oxygenation.

HYPERBILIRUBINEMIA

Definitions

Hyperbilirubinemia (jaundice) is usually caused by an increased bilirubin load in the liver, difficulty clearing the bilirubin from the plasma and impaired conjugation of excretion of bilirubin. Bilirubin is produced from the breakdown of red cell hemoglobin.

Physiological hyperbilirubinemia can be caused due to a combination of the following: Increased RBC volume, decreased survival of fetal RBCs, increased bilirubin from cell breakdown, increased reabsorption of bilirubin from the intestine. Early feeding decreases serum bilirubin by decreasing the reabsorption of bile. This may be caused by increased gut motility. Feeding introduces bacteria into the gut, which contributes to the conversion of bilirubin to urobilin, a substance that cannot be reabsorbed.

Non-physiologic hyperbilirubinemia can occur with ABO/Rh incompatibilities, history of liver disease in the family, maternal illness, labor with trauma or asphyxia and it may also increase with breast-feeding.

Treatment

Hyperbilirubinemia is managed with increased feedings when needed, phototherapy and an exchange transfusion if needed.

Outcome

There is no evidence that healthy term infants without a pathological cause of jaundice are at risk for brain damage, even with levels in the 20-24 mg/dl range. (Maisels and Newman, 1990)

INTRACEREBELLAR HEMORRHAGE

Definition

Intracerebellar hemorrhage results from a primary bleed or extension of the hemorrhage into the cerebellum. This condition is associated with respiratory distress, perinatal asphyxia and prematurity.

Symptoms

The child may present with apnea, bradycardia, decreasing hematocrit and bloody CSF. The three factors of greatest significance include: A large volume of blood present with IVH, increased intracranial pressure and incomplete myelinization of the cerebellum. Incidence 5 to 10% of autopsied neonatal deaths. (Volpe, 1987)

INTRACRANIAL HEMORRHAGE

Definition

Intracranial hemorrhage is a subdural hemorrhage where tears of the cerebral veins and venous sinuses occur with or without lacteration of the dura. It may occur when the infant's head is large compared to size of the birth canal, accompanied with abnormal labor duration, vaginal breech delivery, and malpresentation or difficult instrument-assisted delivery.

Outcome

It usually affects term infants, and the outcome is dependent on the size of the rupture or tear. The infant may develop seizures.

MECONIUM ASPIRATION SYNDROME (MAS)

Definition

Meconium is a mix of epithelial cells and bile salts found in the fetal intestinal tract. With asphyxia in utero, peristalsis is stimulated and relaxation of the anal sphincter occurs, releasing this tar-like stool into the amniotic fluid. Meconium stained fluid is present in 8% to 10% of all pregnancies; severe meconium aspiration is less common.

Complications

Aspiration of the meconium can occur but the risk increases when repeated episodes of severe asphyxia lead to gasping respirations in utero. Complete or partial airway obstruction can occur and a chemical pneumonitis may develop as a result of the aspiration of meconium (possibly due to the bile salts). Asphyxia and chronic hypoxia can predispose the infant to PPHN. Some children with mild meconium aspiration demonstrate difficulty transitioning to textured foods or present with feeding aversion.

Incidence and Symptoms

Meconium aspiration is seldom seen in infants less than 36 weeks gestation. The baby often needs vigorous resuscitation due to central depression. Respiratory distress may range from mild to severe and prolonged. Nail beds and skin appear a stained yellow-green color.

The chest may appear hyperexpanded and complications may include pneumonia, PPHN, BPD, hypoglycemia, hypocalcemia, polycythemia and hyperviscosity. Neurological complications depend on the degree of asphyxia.

Prognosis

Prognosis for infants with mild MAS is generally excellent unless complications of seizures, PPHN or severe asphyxia occur during the course of the disease. In more severe cases, neurological deficits are common and death may occur despite maximum support.

MENINGITIS

Symptoms

Meningitis occurs more frequently during the neonatal period than at any other time. You may see general signs and symptoms of infection and specific CNS symptoms including increased irritability, alterations in consciousness, poor tone, tremors, seizures and bulging fontanel.

Treatment

Prompt antibiotic treatment is needed to optimize outcome. Significant sequelae develop in 20% to 50% of the infants that survive and include motor and mental disabilities, convulsions, hydrocephalus, and hearing loss.

NECROTIZING ENTEROCOLITIS (NEC)

Definition and Incidence

Necrotizing enterocolitis is an acquired disease that affects the GI system, particularly that of premature infants. It is characterized by areas of necrotic bowel in both the small and large intestine. It occurs in 1% to 15% of admissions to the NICU.

Etiology

The cause is unclear but may be related to infections, asphyxia and hypoxia (shunting blood away from the gut to the brain, heart and kidneys so as to protect them), hypertonic feeding (90% to 95% of all infants who get NEC have had enteral feedings) hypovolemia, hypothermia, umbilical line, exchange transfusion, and severe stress or hypotension.

Symptoms

The infant presents with any or all of the following characteristics: Abdominal distention, bilious vomiting, gastric aspirates, bloody stools, lethargy, apnea, bradycardia, temperature instability, hypotension and hypoperfusion.

Treatment

Non-surgical management includes NPO status, gastric decompression, evaluation and correction of hypoxia, acidosis, thrombocytopenia and electrolyte imbalances. Antibiotics, respiratory and circulatory supports are provided as needed. The infant requires careful monitoring of intake and output, blood glucose levels and abdominal girth measuring.

If medical management is not possible or fails, the child should be treated by surgical resection of obvious necrotic bowel. Infant remains NPO until the bowel is functioning and then slow resumption of feedings should be attempted with diluted formula.

Complications

There is a 30% to 40% mortality rate associated with NEC. Gastrointestinal sequelae include strictures, enteric fistulas, diarrhea, and short bowel syndrome with malabsorption problems. The child may also have significant feeding aversion.

PERIVENTRICULAR AND INTRAVENTRICULAR HEMORRHAGE (IVH)

Definition

Periventricular and intraventricular hemorrhage is bleeding in the brain. The germinal matrix is a gelatin like area in the infant's brain that is loaded with nerve cells. This germinal matrix gradually disappears as the nerve cells migrate outward. By term the germinal matrix is almost gone. If the infant is born prematurely, the brain is very susceptible to rupture. IVH causes clots to form. The tissue then dies and forms cystic areas in the brain.

Associated Conditions

IVH is associated with: increasing arterial blood pressure and perinatal asphyxia, prematurity, maternal general anesthesia, low five-minute APGAR scores, acidosis, low birth weight, hypo and hypertension, low hematocrit, respiratory distress requiring mechanical ventilation, PDA ligation and pneumothorax. (Carey, 1983)

Incidence

Incidence of IVH is 32% to 44% of infants with a birth weight less than 1500 grams. In addition, 20% to 30% occur during the first hours of life and the majority occur during the first 72 hours of life. (Bada et al., 1990; Volpe, 1987)

Symptoms

The infant presents with sudden deterioration, oxygen desaturation, bradycardia, metabolic acidosis, hypotonia, shock, hypoglycemia, tense anterior fontanelle and hematocrit significantly decreases. Symptoms of a worsening bleed includes the need for increased ventilatory support, seizures, apnea, full tense fontanels and a decrease in level of consciousness or activity. Bleeds are diagnosed by ultrasound and are no longer classified by grade; however, these classifications may be helpful:

Grade I: Subependymal hemorrhage in the periventricular germinal matrix. Often localized at the Foramen of Monro.
Grade II: Partial filling of lateral ventricles without ventricular dilatation
Grade III: Intraventricular hemorrhage with ventricular dilatation
Grade IV: Parenchymal involvement or extension of blood into the cerebral tissue itself. Can be present to a lesser degree.

Prognosis

Correlation between the severity or extent of involvement and subsequent impairment is not absolute. Because outcomes are so varied, assessment of early symptoms and the practice of purposeful interventions are extremely important. The child may have severe developmental and feeding disorders due to neurological factors.

PERIVENTRICULAR LEUKOMALACIA

Definition

Periventricular leukomalacia is basically a softening of white matter in the brain, and is defined as ischemic-necrotic periventricular white matter. It is typically diagnosed by ultrasound, and 80% to 90% of the cases occur in premature infants. It occurs secondary to inadequate cerebral perfusion, and the outcome is variable based on the location and severity.

Complications

Consequences may include spastic quadriplegia, visual impairment, developmental delays and lower limb weakness. In the older child there may be significant problems with chewing and coordination of the muscles for mastication and swallowing. There may be inconsistencies from day-to-day.

Treatment

Treatment programs should address management strategies for appropriate food consistencies, and supplemental feedings, if needed, for "good" feeding days as well as "bad" feeding days. Oral sensory-motor therapy programs are also recommended for these patients. Motor, speech, language and learning delays may also be present.

Evaluation and Treatment of Pediatric Feeding Disorders: From NICU to Childhood

PERSISTENT PULMONARY HYPERTENSION OF THE NEWBORN (PPHN)

Definition

PPHN is defined as persistence of the cardiopulmonary pathway in the fetus with the dominant feature of high resistance in the pulmonary vessels. This causes obstruction of blood flow through the lungs. The result is right to left shunting of blood through the ductus arteriosus and/or the foramen ovale. PPHN is usually seen in near-term, term or post-term infants with a history of hypoxia or asphyxia at birth. The baby often has low APGAR scores and may have been slow to breath or difficult to ventilate at birth. The baby may have had meconium-stained fluid, nuchal cord or acute blood loss.

Complications

Complications include BPD, air leaks, systemic hypotension, congestive heart failure, kidney damage, hypoglycemia, metabolic acidosis, thrombocytopenia, DIC, hemorrhage, CNS irritability, seizure, edema and abdominal distention.

Treatment

Treatment focuses on correcting hypoxia and acidosis and promoting pulmonary vascular dilation. PPHN mortality is less than 50%. Long-term developmental sequelae need further evaluation. Child may have significant feeding problems.

PLACENTA PREVIA

Definition

Placenta Previa is defined as a placenta that is implanted near the cervix or in varying degrees over the cervix (partial or total). Cervical dilatation at or near term is accompanied by bleeding from the placenta. This occurs in one in 200 deliveries, and in multiparas and older women. It is characterized by bright red, painless vaginal bleeding.

Symptoms

The mother may experience contractions with slight bleeding at first, but bleeding can increase in subsequent episodes. Placenta previa can be diagnosed by ultrasound.

Complications

Potential complications for the mother include: Anemia, hypovolemic shock, endometritis, decreased contractile strength of the lower uterine segment that can lead to postpartum hemorrhage. In some cases, the mother may

54

warrant a hysterectomy. Fetal complications include: Hypoxia, asphyxia, IUGR, premature delivery, developmental anomalies, fetal hemorrhage and death.

Treatment

The mother is placed on bed-rest with no vaginal examinations.

PNEUMONIA

Definition

Pneumonia is an infection of the fetal or newborn lung. Infection may be due to:

- Intrauterine transmission from passage of infecting agent by infection of the fetal membranes.
- Aspiration of meconium or infected amniotic fluid.
- Transplacental transmission.
- Pneumonia may occur in the neonatal period due to pathogens, secondary to a primary disease elsewhere or it may be acquired.
- Intrauterine pneumonia generally follows prolonged rupture of the membranes. Contamination occurs more rapidly if the mother is in active labor. Infective agents may cross the placenta and enter the fetal circulation causing pneumonia.
- Pneumonia may also be caused by bacterial infections, such as Group B beta-hemolytic streptococci, e-coli and staphylococcus aureus or it may be viral from cytomegalovirus, RSV, enterovirus or herpes virus. May also result from aspiration pneumonia.

Symptoms

Infants usually show signs of generalized illness from birth, but signs of illness may be delayed hours to days if the infective fluid is aspirated during delivery. Symptoms include tachypnea, grunting, retractions, cyanosis, hypoxemia and hypercapnia. Other complications include meningitis, cardiac complications, septic shock, disseminated intravascular coagulation (DIC) and persistent pulmonary hypertension.

Treatment

Pneumonia is managed by antibiotic therapy, assisted ventilation, adequate fluid intake and monitoring of temperature, glucose level, and blood pressure.

Prognosis

If severe involvement occurs, shock-like syndrome is seen usually in the first 24 hours of life with recurrent apnea followed by cardiovascular collapse, profound hypoxemia and persistent pulmonary hypertension. Infants with serious bacterial disease at birth are more likely to die regardless of quick and appropriate care, infants with milder bacterial forms are more likely to have a good outcome and for those with viral pneumonia outcome is dependent upon the agent and the overall effects on the patient.

POLYCYTHEMIA

Definition

This is a condition where infants demonstrate an excess in circulating RBC mass. Blood viscosity increases with hematocrit and leads to reduction of blood flow to organs.

Symptoms

May see asymptomatic infants or infants with cyanosis, CNS abnormalities, respiratory distress, tachycardia, congestive heart failure, or hypoglycemia.

Treatment

Treatment includes partial exchange transfusion, desired reduction of hematocrit to less than 60%. Gastrointestinal symptoms of bleeding, poor feeding tolerance, NEC may follow partial exchange. May see increased gross motor, fine motor and speech delays.

POLYHYDRAMINOS

Polyhydraminos is defined as excessive amniotic fluid. Near term, the baby swallows up to half the volume of the amniotic fluid per day. This may also be indicative of an early swallow problem.

PREMATURE RUPTURE OF THE MEMBRANES (PROM)

Premature rupture of the membranes may occur due to infection. The ruptured membranes cause a loss of amniotic fluid. The baby may be able to find a small pocket of amniotic fluid that he or she can continue to breathe. If not, the baby will contract hypoplastic lungs and most likely will have severe respiratory complications.

The Premature Infant: Medical Reference Guide

RESPIRATORY DISTRESS SYNDROME (RDS), OR, HYALINE MEMBRANE DISEASE (HMD)

Definition

RDS/HMD is seen in a large number of premature infants. It is a disorder starting at or soon after birth occurring most frequently in infants with immature lungs. Increasing respiratory difficulty occurs in the first 3 to 6 hours of life and leads to hypoxia and hypoventilation. The infant's lungs lack adequate surfactant, a detergent-like substance that makes the lungs more elastic. The infant takes his first breath, alveoli in the lungs rupture and the lungs are increasingly more difficult to inflate. The infant requires more oxygen and respiratory effort increases.

Precipitating Factors

Precipitating factors include: Prematurity, less than 35 weeks gestation, (the more premature, the more severe the disease), cesarean section without labor, infant of diabetic mother, asphyxia at birth, and twin delivery.

Symptoms

RDS is more common in males than females. The symptoms are progressive and include tachypnea, audible grunting, intercostal and sternal retractions as ventilatory effort increases, nasal flaring and cyanosis due to increasing hypoxemia.

Treatment

Respiratory support and surfactant replacement therapy.

Outcome

Infants with chronic lung disease improve slowly and progressively if they can be maintained infection-free. They commonly have episodes of bronchiolitis and occasionally develop pneumonia during the first years of life. Long-term effects are related to specific complications (BPD, IVH, ROP). Very immature infants typically show more developmental sequelae in later follow up, such as, perceptual problems, and motor delays. The child may have significant feeding problems.

RETINOPATHY OF PREMATURITY

Definition

Retinopathy is eye disease in the premature infant. Normal growth of retinal vessels stop and abnormal new vessels form; 28 to 40 week gestation is an especially active time of development.

57

Contributing Factors

Contributing factors include: medications, high levels of oxygen and exposure to light, prematurity, low birth weight, hypoxia, transfusions, IVH, apnea/bradycardia spells, sepsis, hypercapnia, hypocapnia, PDA, vitamin E deficiency, lactic acidosis and prenatal complications. ROP is classified as stage I, II and III.

Treatment

If more severe, surgery is required. Ninety percent resolve spontaneously with little or no vision loss. Cryotherapy has been shown to decrease the risk of blinding complications by 50%.

SEPSIS

Incidence of sepsis is 1 in 1000 term infants and 1 in 250 premature infants. Group B streptococci and E-coli are responsible for the majority of sepsis cases during the first week of the infant's life. Common sites of infection include the blood, CSF, lungs, and urinary tract. Fifty percent of infants with bacterial sepsis will also present with meningitis.

Clinical findings include hyperthermia or hypothermia, tachypnea/apnea, bradycardia, cyanosis, hypotension, shock, DIC, hepatosplenomegaly, hypoglycemia. There may also be subtle, non-specific signs of temperature lethargy, poor feeding, and observations that the baby is "not acting right."

SUBARCHNOID HEMORRHAGE

Subarchnoid hemorrhage occurs with bleeding of a venous origin in the subarachnoid space. This condition may be precipitated by prematurity, trauma or hypoxia. This bleed is the most common of the neonatal intracranial hemorrhages. Seizure activity may begin day two of life. Hydrocephalus may occur, however, outcome is usually good. (Volpe, 1987)

THROMBOCYTOPENIA

Thrombocytopenia is an acquired disease that causes a significant decrease in the platelet count of the term or premature infant. This results in possible jaundice, bleeding, cranial hemorrhage, anemia and hyperbilirubinemia.

UMBILICAL CORD PROLAPSE

Definition

Umbilical cord prolapse occurs when the umbilical cord falls below the presenting part or is compressed between the presenting part and the pelvis or cervix. The cord may protrude from the vagina or is palpable on vaginal examination. This is a life-threatening event to the fetus. The infant must be delivered quickly.

Predisposing Factors

Predisposing factors include: malposition (transverse lie and breech), pre-term or SGA fetus, multiple infant delivery, polyhydramnios, long umbilical cord, lack of engagement prior to onset of labor and placenta previa.

Outcome

Thirty-five percent of infants die. Mortality increases as increased time elapses between cord prolapse and delivery. If the infant survives he may have fetal anoxia with subsequent long-range neurologic complications. May have severe feeding problems.

Medications

Many medications cause breathing problems and changes, stomach upset or pain. If a child is on multiple medications (for example for seizure disorder, and cardiac), there may be side effects that impact feeding.

Discuss this information with the patient's family and discuss any specific medications your patient is taking. Contact the physician or pharmacist to check for side effects and drug interaction. The following are a few of the medications frequently prescribed for premature infants and medically fragile children.

Aminophylline and Theophylline

These medications are bronchodialators that relax the smooth muscles in the bronchial passages of the lungs. Side effects may include headache, irritability, nausea, vomiting, increased respiratory rate and heart rate, and stomach pain. In more serious reactions, seizures, heart irregularities and breathing difficulties.

Amphetamines

This medication reduces appetite.

Ampicillin

Ampicillin is used to treat infections of the skin, urinary tract and respiratory tract, Group B strep and susceptible E coli. Side effects include diminished urinary output, diarrhea, nausea, vomiting, headache, and pain, and white patches in the mouth. Rare, but serious side effects include rapid, labored breathing, severe abdominal pain and cramping, bloody stools and severe allergic reaction.

Cold Medicines

Many cold medicines can upset the GI tract. This is especially significant for children with special needs.

Decadron

Dacadron is used to increase surfactant and reduce edema. It also helps the baby wean off the vent. Decadron is a corticosteroid.

Dopamine

Dopamine is used to improve cardiac output, blood pressure and urine output from hypotension. Side effects are tachycardia and arrhythmias.

Fentanyl

Fentanyl is a narcotic analgesic taken to relieve pain. Side effects can include drowsiness, breathing problems and physical dependence.

Gentamycin

Gentamycin is a broad-spectrum antibiotic.

Indocin

Indocin is used for closure of the ductus arterious and for prevention of intraventricular hemorrhage.

Lasix

Premature infants organs are also premature and the kidneys have difficulty maintaining water balance. Due to the extra fluid, with BPD the heart does not function as well. Lasix is a diuretic that helps control this but it can be ototoxic. You may have to add sodium chloride to feedings to counteract this, but the sodium chloride may pre-dispose the baby to NEC.

Megestrol, Glucocorticoids and Cyproheptadine

These medications increase appetite.

Phenobarbital

Phenobarbital is a barbiturate, nonselective central nervous system depressant that is primarily used as a sedative hypnotic and also as an anticonvulsant in subhypnotic doses. Side effects include:

- *Nervous system:* agitation, confusion, hyperkinesias, ataxia, CNS depression, nightmares, nervousness, psychiatric disturbance, hallucinations, insomnia, anxiety, dizziness, and thinking abnormality.

- *Respiratory system:* hypoventilation and apnea.
- *Cardiovascular system:* bradycardia, hypotension, and syncope.
- *Digestive system:* nausea, vomiting and constipation.
- *Other reactions may include:* headache, and hypersensitivity reactions (skin rashes, exfoliative dermatitis) fever, and liver damage.

Robinal

Robinal is a medication used to reduce saliva production in children who have problems with secretion management. Robinal reduces, but also thickens secretions, which can increase bacteria levels in the oral cavity. Infants and children need to be carefully assessed and followed closely while on this medication. Robinal dosage needs to be increased over time to maintain results. Tachycardia is a side effect. This drug may not be appropriate for certain patients. In counteraction, there are positional and surgical options to protect the patient from aspiration of saliva.

Vancomycin

Vancomycin is used to treat staph-epi pathogen and septicimia.

CHAPTER FIVE

▲

Evaluation and Treatment of the Newborn: Typical Oral-Motor Development in The Term Infant

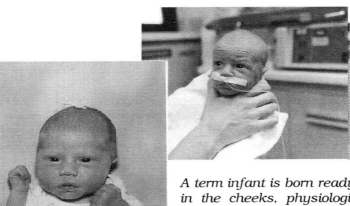

◄ *Preemie baby* ◄

A term infant is born ready to feed with fat pads in the cheeks, physiological flexion, and joint stability. This environment for feeding must be created for the premature infant through swaddling the infant with arms in midline and providing cheek and jaw support during the feeding.

▲ *A term-infant newborn* ▲

Oral Reflexes

The oral reflexes development scale can be used for assessment of infant's feeding skills, justification for waiting until the appropriate time to move to new foods and as a measure of delay. For example, you may state in your report that an 18 month-old infant has the skills of a 6 month-old infant by describing the oral motor movements, intake pattern and amount taken by mouth for your evaluations. This is helpful when calculating months of delay for early intervention or for insurance companies.

Oral reflexes are a major component of the feeding evaluation. If you are evaluating a young premature infant, the baby may be demonstrating a disorganized suckling pattern. Some neonatologists want to start limited nippling attempts with infants as young as 31 weeks gestation. These scales of development help us discuss why we should wait until the baby is 34-36 weeks gestation.

Feeding scales also may help us "predict" a future problem for some infants. Some premature or medically fragile term infants may start having difficulty with feeding after discharge from the hospital, usually at around age 4-6 months when saliva production increases and later when the oral cavity is larger as the fat pads disappear.

Babies with a weak swallow or poor oral motor skills may struggle when teething starts and they may have a hard time managing saliva safely. Feeding also changes, suddenly the baby has a larger area inside the mouth and the baby may have a larger bolus to manage. Some babies develop biting patterns of intake in effort to slow the flow of the bottle at this time.

If you have a baby in your care in the NICU that struggles to feed well, you know that baby is at high risk for additional feeding problems after discharge. Discuss these possibilities with parents and home providers so they can be addressed as soon as they appear. Some babies need a position or nipple change at that time to reduce the flow rate of the feeding; others need a full re-evaluation of the swallow.

The scales also help when it is time to start spoon-feeding attempts. For some reason, this is starting earlier and earlier, with some parents being advised to try spoon as early as two months. We know that tongue protrusion reflex persists until 6 months of age and the baby will reflexively push the food out of the mouth until that reflex is integrated. With a typical baby this is not that major of an issue, however, with a preemie or infant with tone issues, spoon-feeding can place a child at very high risk for aspiration.

Remember children need a foundation of feeding skills. For example, if the child does not demonstrate jaw stability, it will be difficult to create effective lip seal and push a thicker consistency bolus back for efficient swallowing. All the pieces need to be there or compensated for with external support or careful positioning strategies.

How to Evaluate Oral Reflexes

When you assess oral reflexes, use latex free, no powder gloves and make sure your fingernails are short. Use your pinky finger to gently stroke down the lip to see if the root reflex is present. You may have to stimulate the reflex several times with a premature or medically fragile term infant. When the baby opens the mouth, place your finger (pad side, not nail side) on lower lip and gently move to the anterior tongue and follow with a slight stroke back toward the lip. Repeat as needed. If you do not elicit a reflex, turn your finger pad up against the hard palate. Press firmly and wait. Many times this firm pressure input will elicit a sucking pattern. Is the suck coordinated? Does the baby alternate between biting and sucking? What is his endurance level? Is the tongue cupped around your finger? Where is the tongue at rest?

Once in the mouth, gently move your finger to the side of the tongue and apply pressure or rub the surface. This will stimulate the transverse tongue reflex. This one persists throughout life and is the one that is elicited when we visit the dentist! This reflex should be the same on both sides. Move to the gum ridge and put pressure by pressing down on the gums, you should feel a bite of equal pressure on both sides. A very strong bite response is not normal and can indicate a tonic bite reflex. Ask the nurse about the gag and save this for last. Note where the gag triggers and how easily it is elicited. Some babies do not gag until you are deep in the pharynx or they do not gag at all. That tells you that the sensory feedback in the pharynx may be very poor. If the baby doesn't feel your finger, will he feel liquid in his throat as he is feeding? Single bolus swallows via pacifier and syringe, using chilled formula may be your best option in starting therapy with these patients.

SUCKLING

Suckling emerges at 13 to 24 weeks gestational age and persists until approximately 32 weeks gestation. Characterized by a disordered pattern of sucking bursts and pauses. This pattern is then replaced by a more stable pattern of rhythmical sucking and swallowing by 34 to 36 weeks gestation. The strength of the suck also increases with anatomic and neurological maturation. For the first months of life, the non-nutritive pattern of tongue movement is to extend and retract the tongue, allowing the nipple to be drawn into the mouth to initiate feeding. At 3 to 4 months of age the infant begins to develop lateral tongue movements that allow for some degree of bolus manipulation.

SUCKING

Develops between 6 and 9 months of age. This is the second type of intake pattern characterized by rhythmical sustained movement, but now the tongue raises and lowers in a strong pumping-like motion. The infant now has a more sophisticated pattern of bolus formulation and can remove soft-textured food from a spoon. The oral cavity begins to remodel and enlarge as the buccal fat pads resorb, a masticatory surface is created as the alveolar ridges, and later the teeth form. Jaw movement is decreased and lips are more firmly approximated, providing the stability and intra-oral pressure to propel thicker consistencies of food through the oral cavity and back for initiation of the swallow. Increasingly mature patterns of mastication develop between 6 and 8 months of age. By 12 month, sucking patterns are minimized and children generally transition to cup drinking as they no longer use the sucking pattern. (Rudolph)

GAG

A gag emerges at 26 to 27 weeks gestational age and persists throughout life for safety reasons.

PHASIC BITE

A phasic bite emerges at 28 weeks and is characterized by rhythmical closing and opening of the jaw in response to stimulation of the gums. Integrates at 9 to 12 months of age.

TRANSVERSE TONGUE REFLEX

A transverse tongue reflex emerges at 28 weeks gestational age and is characterized by movement of the tongue to the side of stimulation. Persists through life.

TONGUE PROTRUSTION

Evident at term. Characterized by protrusion of the tongue when stimulated anteriorly. Integrated at 4-6 months of age. Introduction of baby foods prior to six months results in a "battle" against this reflex as the spoon continually stimulates tongue protrusion.

ROOT REFLEX

A root reflex emerges at 32 weeks and is characterized by head turning to the side of the cheeks or corners of the mouth. Integrates at 3 to 6 months of age. Should be elicited during breast or bottle-feeding by stimulating the lower lip, rather than on either cheek or side of the mouth. (Lawrence)

Feeding Skills by Age and Volume Per Feeding

The following combines research on feeding development from different authors from speech pathology as well as information from dietitians and physicians to develop a quick, multi-source reference guide for the therapist.

Age of child	Number of feedings per day	Volume per feeding
0-1 months old	6-8 feedings of breastmilk or formula	2-5 ounces Breastfed baby should nurse 8-12 times per day or on demand, at least 5-10 minutes on each side. Baby should produce six wet diapers per day.
2-3 months old	4-7 feedings of breastmilk or formula	5-7 ounces
3-4 months old	4-7 feedings of breastmilk or formula	6-8 ounces
4-6 months	4-6 feedings of breastmilk or formula. Introduce iron-fortified baby cereal at 6-months. Feed only one new cereal per week to check for sensitivity. Do not add salt or sugar to cereal.	6-8 ounces

NEWBORN TO THREE MONTHS

Suckling continues at this time. Look for coordinated suck-swallow-breathe sequences initially. The usual volume of milk taken in during each suck by a term infant is approximately 0.2 mL, requiring 300 sucking and swallowing events to consume 60 mL, which a normal infant can consume in approximately 5 minutes. The pre-term infant generates lower suction pressures, with smaller amounts of milk per suck. (Mathew, Belan and Thoppil)

At three months, the baby may sequence twenty or more sucks from the breast or bottle, breathing follows sucking with no discernible pauses when hungry. Pauses for breathing are infrequent.

The baby starts to develop primitive tongue lateralization skills. Occasional coughing or choking may indicate poor coordination of the suck-swallow-breathe sequence.

Skills are not appropriate for soft/pureed foods. If soft or pureed foods are presented, the infant uses a primitive suckle-swallow response to move food into the pharynx. Tongue protrusion reflex is stimulated and food is pushed out of the mouth. Periodic choking, gagging or vomiting can occur.

FOUR TO SIX MONTHS

The baby uses long sequences of sucking, swallowing and breathing with breast or bottle. If the baby is not gaining weight adequately, you may need to concentrate the formula (follow dietitian recommendations), add blenderized cereal to the feeding and/or increase frequency of feedings. Be careful though that the baby has enough time between feedings to rest, digest food and feel hunger at the next feeding.

Do not slit nipples. A slit nipple does not remain consistent and with use the cut can continue to widen. This can significantly impact the feeding and there is a risk of aspiration from high flow rate. There are high flow nipples on the market and products made for thickened feedings. The nipple hole size remains consistent and the baby is much safer with these products. Refer to nipple comparison chart for additional information.

The dietitian and physician should carefully monitor the infant's weight and intake patterns.

Baby food should be introduced at six months or when motor skills support spoon-feeding attempts. The child must have head control and be able to sit with support or have special positioning recommendations from an occupational or physical therapist.

The tongue now shows an extension-retraction pattern or simple protrusion between the teeth or gums. Food is not pushed out of the mouth by the tongue, although minor losses of food may continue intermittently.

Cup Drinking

A four-month-old infant lacks appropriate skills for cup drinking. Introduce cup at 6 months. When the infant is taking liquids from a cup, he may have continuous sucks followed by periods of uncoordinated swallowing. Much of the liquid is lost. Larger mouthfuls may result in choking or coughing.

Suckling pattern with extension-retraction motions of the tongue are observed during drinking or as the cup is offered or removed. Wide jaw excursions are common.

Reflex Development

The sucking reflex emerges. This second type of intake develops and is characterized by rhythmical, sustained movement with the tongue elevating and lowering in a strong pumping-like motion.

Changes

Jaw movement is decreased and lips are more firmly approximated. This change prepares the infant to build adequate intra-oral negative pressure to successfully propel thicker consistencies of food through the oral cavity and back into the pharynx for swallowing. Tongue protrusion reflex is also typically integrated at 4-6 months of age.

Age of child	Feedings per day	Volume per feeding
6-9 months old	3-4 feedings breastmilk or formula per day	1/4-1/2 cup servings of baby food. As child approaches 8-9 months, try small tastes of mashed potatoes and gravy, vanilla custard style yogurt, scrambled egg yolks, applesauce or oatmeal.
9-12 months old	3-4 servings of 6-8 ounces of breastmilk or formula per day	Cheese/Yogurts: 1/2 ounce or 1/2 cup serving. Grains: Offer 2-3 times per day in two to four tablespoons of iron fortified baby cereal, 1/2 slice of bread or two crackers Fruit: Three ounces of juice or 2 servings of three to four tablespoons of fresh or pureed fruit Vegetables: Offer 2-3 times per day in three to four tablespoon size servings Meats: Offer two times per day in 3-4 tablespoon size servings

SIX TO NINE MONTHS

Cup Drinking

The baby may struggle with the transition to cup at 6 months. A soft spout cup may help with this transition. Make sure the 6 month old can handle the flow rate of the cup. At 9 months the infant uses long sequences of continuous sucks during cup drinking. The baby may still have difficulty coordinating sucks with swallowing and breathing. Although longer coordinated sucks are possible, the baby usually takes up to three sucks before stopping or pulling away to breathe.

Semi-solids

With semi-solids, you may see an up-down sucking pattern of sucking. Simple tongue protrusion is noted between the teeth or gums. Some extension-retraction movement of the tongue may also continue intermittently.

Changes

The phasic bite reflex becomes integrated at this time to allow for a more mature chewing pattern to emerge.

NINE TO TWELVE MONTHS

Cup Drinking

When taking liquids from a cup, swallowing follows sucking with no clear pause. The baby can sequence at least three suck-swallows when thirsty. Some coughing and choking may occur if liquid flows too fast.

Soft Solids

Baby swallows soft solids with intermittently elevated tongue-tip position. This tongue pattern may alternate with a pattern of simple tongue protrusion. True tongue lateralization is now emerging.

Changes

Swallows ground, mashed, or chopped soft foods with small lumps. The child uses an intermittently elevated tongue tip, but may have tongue protrusion. No extension-retraction movements now occur during swallowing. When biting, the child uses a controlled, sustained bite on a soft cookie. May not be able to sustain biting on a hard cookie and may revert back to a phasic bite or sucking.

Quantity

- Formula or breastmilk continues at 3-4 servings of 6-8 ounces per feeding.
- Cheese or yogurt can be offered in portions of 1/2 oz or 1/2 cup.
- Grains can be offered 2-3 times per day as 2-4 T. of iron fortified baby cereal, 1/2 slice of bread or two crackers.
- Fruit should be offered in 2 servings of 3-4 T. or 3 ounces of juice.
- Vegetables should be offered 2-3 times per day in servings of 3-4 tablespoons.
- Meats should be offered 2 times per day in 3-4 T. servings.

THE OLDER CHILD: TWELVE TO FIFTEEN MONTHS

Cup Drinking

When taking liquids from a cup, swallowing follows sucking with no pause. Pattern is well coordinated and coughing/choking rarely occurs. The baby can now sequence at least three suck-swallows while drinking one ounce or more without a major pause.

Changes

Upper incisors are used to clean the lower lip as it draws inward. Uses a sucking pattern with spoon, may bite on the spoon, but the phasic bite reflex has been integrated and is not present. Munching pattern continues with improved tongue lateralization. The child begins to self-feed, develops pincer grasp and holds his own cup.

Food types

Whole milk can begin at 12 months and continue until child is two years old. At fifteen months child is given liquids and introduced to coarsely chopped table foods, including easily chewed meat. Watch the child for signs of readiness and add condiments or gravies to more challenging foods. Consider alternating solids with purees if child is not completely clearing the oral cavity between bites.

Textures and Tastes

Offer a variety of foods that are soft and expose the child to mixed textures, such as: pudding with crumbled graham cracker, fork mashed chicken pot pie (meat when closer to 15 months), spaghetti, scrambled eggs with cheese, pancake with blueberries or bananas, finely ground meat and gravy and fruit yogurts.

Respect your child's likes and dislikes; offer rejected foods again a few days later. Tastes are developing.

Quantity

Feed the toddler 3 snacks a day. Juice should be limited to only 4 ounces per day. Children should only drink water, milk and juice until age two. Do not allow child to carry a bottle or cup of milk/juice around during the day. This can lead to "grazing" patterns; continuous eating or drinking small amounts through the day that dampen or inhibit appetite. This pattern of intake does not promote adequate nutrition. Avoid soda and tea and sports drinks. Children usually take one good (by parent's definition) meal a day. Appetite is highly variable; if weight gain is adequate, do not be alarmed.

EIGHTEEN MONTHS

Changes

Sucking pattern with external jaw stabilization obtained by biting down on the edge of the cup. The upper lip is closed on the edge of the cup, providing a better seal for drinking. Tongue does not protrude from the mouth or rest beneath the cup. Minimal wide jaw excursions up-down or backward-forward patterns of movement may be observed if stabilization is not used. The baby now demonstrates excellent hand to mouth skills.

Semi-Solids

With semi-solids uses tongue tip elevation intermittently or consistently for swallowing. Simple tongue protrusion may occur during swallowing, however, there is no extension-retraction movements of the tongue.

Rotary chewing skills are noted with solid foods and increased tongue lateralization results in more effective handling of food. The child swallows solid foods with easy lip closure as needed. No loss of saliva or food. Tongue tip elevation used for swallowing. Some simple tongue protrusion may continue during swallowing.

Solids

The child uses a controlled, sustained bite on a hard cookie. May use overflow or associated arm or leg movements during biting. She child may pull the head backward into slight extension to assist with the bite.

Food Types

Child is given liquids and coarsely chopped table foods, including most soft meats and some raw vegetables if skills are appropriate. Other food ideas include: fruit yogurts, cereal, pasta, rice, muffins, rolls, crackers, fish, turkey, peas, corn, and baked sweet potatoes.

TWENTY-FOUR MONTHS

Cup Drinking

With cup drinking the child uses a sucking pattern and active internal jaw stabilization without biting the edge of the cup. Internal stabilization occurs most of the time during drinking sequences of more than two sucks. Slight up-down jaw motions or holding the edge of the cup with the teeth may also occur.

Soft Solids

The child should now swallow soft solids with no loss of food or saliva. He uses tongue tip elevation for swallowing. No tongue protrustion at this stage of development.

Solids

The child swallows solid foods, including those with a combination of textures, with easy lip closure as needed. No loss of food or saliva, skillfully swallows foods that have a combination of textures.

Changes

Tongue tip elevation is used for swallowing. Tongue is used in a free sweeping motion to clean food from the upper or lower lips. Tongue elevation and depression are independent of jaw movement. Skillful tongue tip action may be present. Slight lateral movement of the jaw may occur. The child uses a controlled, sustained bite while keeping the head in midline when food is presented for biting on both sides of the mouth. The child is able to grade the opening of the jaw when biting through foods of various thicknesses. Child presents with mature chewing and drinking skills.

Quantity

- Four servings of milk
- Six servings of grains
- Two servings of fruit
- Three servings of vegetables
- Two servings of meat
- Limit juice to 4 ounces per day

A Word About Juice

Caution parents about the calories in drinks such as Kool-Aid, juice, soda or sweetened tea. Many parents do not think about the effects these sugared liquids have an appetite or how they may contribute either to failure to thrive or early obesity. Some children like to carry their cup with them and filling it multiple times per day can result in liquid intake up to 80 ounces per day. In some children this will result in poor appetite and poor weight gain and in others will result in excessive weight gain. Obesity can lead to diabetes, heart disease or multiple health issues. Many times the juice cup is the culprit. Limit juice to 4 ounces per day. Water should be given between structured meals and snacks. Avoid grazing on foods or liquids.

Bottle Feeding Guidelines

- Ready to use formulas are more convenient, but do not contain fluoride. Powdered formula and liquid concentrate are more economical and should be mixed with sterile water. Some infants with hypersensitivity will reject powdered formulas after having ready to use in the hospital. Be consistent and use the formula your doctor/dietitian has recommended, do not buy the formula that is on sale week to week.

- Formula may be given at room temperature or lukewarm, but should be stored in the refrigerator after it is mixed or the container is opened.

- Offer 3 oz of formula when you get home from the hospital, do not force your baby to finish the bottle. Do not save left over formula for the next feeding.

- When increasing volume of feedings do so gradually. When the newborn baby completely finishes 2 or more feedings, increase the amount by 1/2 ounce. Repeat this practice as the baby grows and requires additional volume of formula or breastmilk.

- Burp the baby in the middle and at the end of each feeding. Infant's appetites may vary day to day, but if poor feedings persist over a 24-hour period, call your physician.

- Never prop a baby with a bottle. Hold the baby semi-upright during the feeding. This decreases the risk of "positional otitis media." Because the infant's head is elevated, sucking and swallowing propel the milk with a peristaltic motion to the stomach in a process that protects the Eustachian tube from entry of milk. This synchronous motion also minimizes choking and regurgitation. (Lawrence)

Infant Formula Guide

Reflux is a mechanical problem and is not influenced by the type of formula used. Many infants go through "formula roulette" when they have problems with spitting/vomiting and frequent formula change is not necessary. Specialized formulas are expensive and should only be used for children that meet the criteria described below. Caution parents to use one formula consistently. *Review preparation of formulas with patients' families especially if concentrated formula (high caloric density) is recommended. Seek recommendations from a pediatric dietitian or gastroenterologist. Parent instruction must be completed by the dietitian or physician to concentrate feedings.*

STANDARD COW'S MILK FORMULAS

These types of formula may be recommended for infants who have achieved a weight of 2-2.5kg and are not receiving their mother's milk. This formula has had removal of butterfat and some of the proteins. Vegetable oil and additional carbohydrates have been added in the form of lactose. Standard formula has 20 kcal/oz. These formulas can be mixed to a higher caloric density of 24kcal/oz under supervision of a dietitian. Examples: Similac, and Enfamil.

SOY FORMULAS

These formulas are not recommended for feeding preterm infants because of the decreased bioavailability of calcium and phosphorus in these products. Hypophosphatemia has been reported in full-term infants. Preterm infants are at an increased risk for alteration in bone mineralization and the incidence of rickets is higher in this population. Soy formulas have vegetable oil and carbohydrates in the form of sucrose. This formula also contains higher levels of soy protein. Soy is not as easily absorbed as the protein in cow's milk formulas. A baby needs the right amount of protein for normal growth but not so much that it taxes the kidneys. Soy formula is often used with babies who have rare conditions such as Galactosemia or Lactose Deficiency. Refer to AAP's position on use of soy formula with infants. Examples: Isomil, Prosoybee.

HYDROLYZED WHEY-BASED FORMULA

Carnation Good Start is the only commercial partially-hydrolysated whey formula on the market. This formula can be used with VLBW infants in place of standard cow's milk formula with the same caveats. In this product, the whey fraction of cow's milk protein has been broken down by enzyme hydrolysis to yield smaller protein fractions, making it less allergenic than the whole proteins of regular formulas. However, Good Start is not a casein hydrolysate and thus maintains the potential to provoke serious allergic response in sensitive infants.

CASEIN HYDROLYSATE (ELEMENTAL) FORMULAS

Casein hydrolysate formulas may be used with VLBW infants who have special needs. They tend to be expensive and should only be used when truly needed. Nutramigen, Pregestimil and Alimentum are formulas based on a hypoallergenic protein source consisting of amino acids and small peptides. They are useful when there has been damage to an infant's GI tract from a viral or bacterial infection or complications of prematurity such as NEC. An immature or damaged GI tract is permeable to foreign proteins, predisposing the infant to an allergic condition. Use of casein hydrolysates may improve digestion and allow for mucosal healing and recovery of function. This would allow a progressive return to more standard formulas.

These products may also be appropriate if an infant presents with malabsorption. With significant fat malabsorption, Pregestimil or Alimentum may be the products of choice because about half of the fat is provided by MCT (medium chain triglycerides) which do not require the normal fat digestive pathways. It has been suggested that these products might be useful in times of acute GI infection as well.

AMINO ACID-BASED FORMULA

There are infants who have difficulty with even casein hydrolysate formulas and may require amino acid-based formulas. Neocate and Elecare are the only formulas of this type on the market at this time. These products are designed for infants who have severe milk protein intolerance.

FOLLOW-UP FORMULAS

Reportedly designed for older babies with less fat and more protein and minerals. No documented advantage to using this formula over standard formulas.

Introduction of Semi-Solid and Solid Foods

Following are general recommendations (unless the physician tells you otherwise):

- Least allergenic foods are offered first and in this order: infant rice cereal, strained vegetables, fruits, juices and meats.
- Serve only one new food every 7 days so you can watch for allergic reactions such as skin rash, diarrhea, constipation or vomiting.
- Begin with strained foods and increase the texture as baby develops. Do not add foods to the bottle, baby needs to develop a chewing pattern and he may develop an aversion to the spoon later when it is introduced.
- Mixed infant dinners and desserts have less nutritional value. Buy single ingredient foods.
- Use a small bowl for baby food feedings. Feeding out of the jar is not recommended because saliva from the baby's mouth can spoil uneaten food quickly.
- Salts and sweets are not recommended.
- Do not offer cow's milk until one year of age. Whole milk is recommended when milk is introduced.

Spoon Feeding Guidelines

General recommendations:

- Do not start spoon-feeding until the baby is six-months old. At that time the infant has the skills to control the thicker consistency food, form and propel a bolus back for swallowing. Effective spoon-feeding is closely related to the infant's ability to sit up and control the head and shoulder girdle.
- A pacifier can be used as the first spoon or between bites to help the infant clear the oral cavity. Some infants may need tastes on pacifier and teethers before any attempts with spoon. The spoon can also be used as a teether to help the child get used to the texture and feel of it. Soft bowl spoons from Sassy and Gerber may also be very effective with children who gag easily.
- Rest the spoon on the lower lip and allow the baby to suck the tastes off the spoon. Do not immediately remove the spoon from the mouth, the baby will use the spoon as a point of stability and as a substitute for the nipple while they are learning the new skill.
- Do not scrape food off on the alveolar ridge or put the spoon deep in the mouth.
- Some babies with sensory issues cannot handle the consistency and texture of rice cereal for their first spoon feedings. Some infants respond best to smooth and strong flavors of baby food fruit alone. Try to follow the rules of vegetables first when possible, but take into account the complete picture of the infant you are working with and make decisions for the individual child. Remember that some children with significant sensory or neurological history may have altered taste patterns.

Cup Drinking

Make sure the child has the postural stability to support the move to cup drinking. Newborns without medical issues can attempt cup at 6 months and will still show reduced coordination of suck/swallow/breathe sequence at 9 months. This is normal. Preemies are often not ready to drink from a cup at 6 months, judge the infant's readiness by assessing head, shoulder girdle and trunk strength and stability, respiratory status (may be easier than bottle with some infants) and bolus formulation and control.

- Put a very small amount of formula or breastmilk in the cup initially so the infant is not overwhelmed by the liquid flow rate. You do not want the baby to develop an aversive response to the cup.
- The Avent Soft Spout Cup is an excellent product due to the soft spout that seals the mouth well. The infant who is used to the texture of a pliable nipple, may transition easier to a soft spout than to a hard plastic spout. With some children, the therapist can dip the

spout in the smallest tastes of baby food just to help the patient get used to the feel of it and begin the transition to cup drinking. A baby needs time to become familiar with utensils and spouts without the pressure of taking food or liquid off of them. Children learn about their world by mouthing. The spout can also be chilled and offered as a teether at first for very sensitive children.

- If thickened formula is required blenderized rice cereal can be added at 1/2 tsp per ounce or more as needed. Thick-It can be used for water and is not the only method of thickening for all liquids. Thick-It does not remain consistent over time and can alter taste. See alternatives below.

- If children older than one year require thickening of liquids consider the following alternatives to Thick It or Thick'em Up:

Milk or Pediasure thickened with pudding packs, ice cream and/or *Carnation Instant Breakfast Powder* are great calorie boosters. A standard recipe is 4 ounces of milk to 6-8 ounces of pudding.

Juice thickened with orange sherbet or pureed fruit (applesauce in apple juice). Standard recipe 4 ounces of juice to 8 ounces of puree, increase as needed.

Orange Juice/Orange Sherbet/7up works well to clear the pharynx as it does not coat the throat and is great for oral alerting. Standard recipe is 4 ounces of orange juice, 6 ounces of sherbet and 1/4 cup 7up.

Yogurt or fruit smoothies (add Danimals Drinkable Yogurt, Yoplait Custard Style Yogurt, fruit, CIB powder in blender).

Infant Appetite

Appetite is controlled by hunger and satiety centers in the hypothalamus. Hunger results from an integration of a variety of sensory inputs (taste, smell, and vision), limbic and cortical inputs (mood), and visceral feedback (noxious experiences, gastric volume, substrates, and hormones). The factors that impact appetite in infants vary depending on experience Infants have preferences for sweet formula until age 4 months and then prefer salty. (Beauchamp, Cowart, Moran)

Even minor changes in human milk induced by maternal alcohol or garlic ingestion can alter milk intake by the infant. (Mennella, Beauchamp) Infants who are not nurtured reduce food intake. (Gagan, Cupoli, Watkins) Also, see food reductions in children with chronic debilitating diseases by Rudolph.

Infant/child appetite is also related to weight gain. Children who fall off the scale or below the third percentile may develop childhood anorexia. Nasogastric feedings in weak, lethargic children or supplemental feedings may be needed to help the child regain appetite and improve weight gain.

CHAPTER SIX
▲
Breastfeeding

Therapist Chat

Breastfeeding is supposed to easy and natural, right? Breastfeeding is actually the first learning experience a mother and her infant will share and at times it comes with difficulty. Engorgement, sore nipples, the myth of insufficient milk supply, and difficulty with latch on only name a few common breastfeeding hurdles.

Children who breastfeed can present with similar oral motor and swallowing difficulties as their bottle fed peers, but specialized understanding of breastfeeding is required to successfully treat this population. While working with an infant who is breastfed it is essential to have an understanding of the mechanics of breastfeeding, the pros and cons to the tools available, and have an appreciation of the importance of positioning for adequate latch on. We encourage you to train with a Certified Lactation Consultant to gain an overall appreciation for working with the breastfed infant. Making rounds in the birth center as well as seeing outpatients with the Lactation Consultant will provide you with a variety of experiences. Trainings are also available to become a Certified Lactation Consultant.

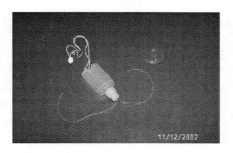

A supplemental nursing system of SNS (left) and nipple shield (right) are devices used to assist mothers who are experiencing breastfeeding difficulties. A SNS is used to provide a supplement of pumped breastmilk or formula while the infant is nursing. Supplemental feeding at the breast instead of with a bottle provides a mother with stimulation from the infant's sucking to improve her milk production. A nipple shield may be necessary if the infant is seeking increased proprioceptive input in order to latch on. The shield also assists with breastfeeding if firm input is necessary to achieve correct tongue positioning for a retracted tongue.

Case Example: Grace

HISTORY

Molly and Ben were expecting their first baby. They prepared for their child's arrival by reading the right books, attending prenatal, Lamaze and parenting classes; they had everything ready for the new baby. Molly only had a six-week maternity leave, however, she was reducing her hours and Ben was taking one day a week off for the next month to be with the baby. Finally, the big day arrived. Molly had a remarkably easy delivery for a first baby. They had a little girl and named her Grace. Molly had decided to breastfeed. Grace breastfed well and the next few weeks were good ones for the family.

At her first well baby check-up the doctor asked Molly what her plans were for feeding her baby after she returned to work. Molly was a surgery nurse and would not be able to take breaks to feed her baby. She might be in surgery for 12-14 hours at times. She wasn't working as many days as before the baby, but she decided to pump her breast milk and feed Grace with a bottle. The doctor told her to attempt bottle a few weeks before returning work. Week four of her leave, Molly tried to feed Grace with a variety of different bottles. Grace, perfect, content, easygoing little Grace screamed in frustration. She kept turning toward Molly, searching for the breast. She opened her mouth wide and didn't know what to do with the bottle. When the nipple touched her tongue, she gagged and Molly was afraid she was going to vomit. Molly felt the first flickers of fear. Why was this so hard? Was something wrong? She only had two weeks left. She called her mother. Her mother told her that Ben should try to feed her, because when Molly was around Grace wanted to nurse. That made sense, so Molly was less anxious. Molly felt foolish, but she wasn't thinking like a nurse and she couldn't analyze Grace like a patient. Later that evening, Ben attempted the bottle. Grace still screamed and turned away, but finally settled down and took three ounces with an awkward suck. Molly noticed that Grace had spilled a lot of milk down her chin as she was drinking from the bottle. However, they had managed the first feeding. Ben put Grace over his shoulder to burp her and she vomited the entire feeding down his back. This was the beginning of a pattern of long crying spells, bottle refusals, and vomiting and poor feedings over the next two weeks. Molly had received many "tips" to help Grace take to the bottle, including: using a red hospital nipple for premature infants; cutting the nipple for a faster flow rate; switching her to formula because the baby was "probably having problems tolerating her breastmilk"; and she was also encouraged to stop confusing the baby by breast and bottle feeding. Molly was now in a panic. It was time to return to work, Grace had not gained weight well over the past two weeks, had developed an ear infection and feedings were improving, but continued to be a daily struggle. Molly fed Grace frequently because of her fear of losing weight. The vomiting also increased significantly so Molly decided to try formula for a feeding. Grace was so gassy and miserable that she cried all night. Molly considered a trip to the emergency room because Grace screamed like she was in pain. Molly and Ben were bewildered and upset that something was wrong with their baby. Vomiting now occurred with almost every feeding. Molly's milk supply started to decrease and she was terrified that her baby would not have enough of her breast milk and would not be able to take the bottle well enough to meet her nutritional needs. Molly again called her doctor; they needed help.

Breastfeeding

EVALUATION AND TREATMENT

Molly, Ben and Grace were referred to a pediatric feeding team. Team members included the pediatric gastroenterologist, dietitian, speech therapist/feeding specialist, occupational therapist, pediatric nurse and lactation consultant. The team listened to the complaint, reviewed the family medical history and assessed feeding. The following recommendations were made:

1. The gastroenterologist explained reflux to Molly and Ben. They were told that the lower esophageal sphincter opened and closed randomly with young babies. Spitting was a normal part of infancy and the physician explained how most infants improve at six months and often grow out of it by one year of age. The family was instructed to keep Molly upright and in a position that did not put pressure on the abdomen 20-30 minutes after the feeding. Rice cereal, 1/2 teaspoon per bottle, was added to the feedings in order to reduce the risk of reflux. Medications were not used to treat reflux at this time. Diagnostic treatment with other measures from the team would be explored and Grace was scheduled for a follow-up visit in two weeks.

2. The feeding specialist explained to Molly and Ben that bottle and breastfeeding were two completely different acts. When bottle-feeding a baby has to actually draw the milk out of the nipple with two forces, compression and suction. The baby uses the lips to draw milk out of the bottle. With breastfeeding the breast tissue is drawn in deep, the milk lets down and fills the mouth. The baby closes the lips to *stop* the flow of milk. That is why Grace opened her mouth wide around the bottle nipple. She was having a hard time learning how to suck. Molly was given a therapeutic pacifier, shaped like the bottle nipple to teach Grace to suck better from a bottle. It is a fallacy that babies should not have a pacifier. There are many, many benefits *when a pacifier is used correctly.* Grace needed to figure out how to suck with compression and suction. They dipped the pacifier in breast milk and Molly and Ben were given exercises to stimulate Grace's suck reflex and to strengthen it.

3. Grace was also on the wrong bottle due to her special feeding needs. Standard bottles did not seal her mouth well and she was taking an excessive amount of air with her feedings. Grace was munching and biting on the nipple instead of sucking well. She needed a nipple that sealed her lips well and extended farther into her mouth that she could cup her tongue around. The Dr. Brown Bottle with the Y-cut nipple was selected for a trial of use at home and 1/2 teaspoon of rice cereal per ounce of formula was added to the feedings. The Y-cut nipple was used so the feedings could be thickened and still pass easily through the nipple and also the cereal could help add density to the feeding to reduce spitting and improve weight gain. This patented bottle was selected as it contains an internal venting system and separates air from the liquid. It was felt that air trapping was contributing to Grace's vomiting. No

79

vacuum was created with this bottle so less air was passed to the middle ear. Grace also had a history of ear infections, so this bottle was the best option for her needs.

4. The feeding specialist, lactation consultant and occupational therapist assessed the position Grace was held in during feedings. For breastfeeding, Grace was placed in a cross-football hold. Molly was instructed to give Grace plenty of support to her body and to slightly stretch her out across her body. This would allow Grace to breathe well and to reduce the pressure on her stomach as she was feeding. For bottle feedings, Grace was firmly swaddled with a blanket around her hips and less firmly around her shoulders. Swaddling calmed her and supported her body well so the muscles of her face could work efficiently to take the bottle.

5. Molly was seen by the lactation consultant who put her on a pumping schedule every two hours to increase her milk supply. Molly had extended her maternity leave to 12 weeks due to Grace's feeding problems. The goal was to build up the milk supply by pumping and to build up Molly's supply of frozen breast milk. Molly was cautioned that excessive stress could reduce her milk supply. She was given a progressive relaxation tape with soothing music to listen to while she pumped or fed Grace. Molly was followed by lactation weekly to monitor her milk production.

6. The lactation specialist and feeding specialist found in their discussions with Molly that she truly wanted to continue breastfeeding, but was fearful Grace would continue to experience difficulty with bottle-feeding. Treatment focused on continuing both methods of feeding; as ongoing breastfeeding was desired by the family and would help maintain Molly's milk supply.

7. The family kept feeding logs and sent them to the dietitian. The feeding specialist monitored Grace's progress with the Dr. Brown Bottle. Grace was also seen for weekly weight checks.

8. The team also suggested a foam wedge and Tucker sling to put Grace on her stomach and keep her in a semi-upright position to reduce the risk of vomiting. The feeding specialist and occupational therapist instructed the family how to safely use the wedge and sling and cautioned them regarding the risk of SIDS in prone. Grace was to be supervised while on the wedge.

9. The family was also instructed in Kangaroo Care, skin-to-skin contact, with the baby held to either parent's bare chest and covered by a blanket after feedings. This would keep Grace upright and was very calming for her. K-care also helps improve the supply of breastmilk that the mother produces. This family had missed much of the quality time together that they needed during the maternity leave, so this was also seen as a great

bonding time. From a neurodevelopmental perspective, the skin-to-skin contact helped Grace remain calm and gave her input to her body.

10. Social work service assisted Molly with applications for Child and Family Leave Act coverage to protect her position at work. Daycare options were also investigated and videotaped feedings were provided to daycare workers to demonstrate proper feeding technique. This significantly decreased stress level on the family.

RESULT

Grace had less spitting and colicky behaviors and slept better. She eventually fed very well at the breast as well as with the Dr. Brown Bottle. No anti-reflux medications were needed. Molly's milk supply increased dramatically with scheduled pumping. Weight gain stabilized and incidence of ear infections decreased. Molly was able to return to work after a 12-week maternity leave.

Nipple Confusion Fact or Fiction?
(Neifert, Lawrence and Seacat)

Breast and bottle-feeding are very different methods of feeding. Nipples on the market vary dramatically in texture, flow rate and size. Nipple confusion is a broad, easy term that does not encourage the therapist to define what is occurring with the infant or the mother. Many infants are actually experiencing subtle feeding problems and while feeding at breast, especially if the mother has a good milk supply, (the baby simply swallows fast flow of milk) these feeding problems may be masked until the mother tries to introduce the bottle. Other infants are actually experiencing flow rate confusion, bottle-to-bottle confusion, positioning confusion or reacting to different sensory input between bottle- and breast-feeding.

Medical research defines two types of "nipple confusion" to describe the impact of artificial nipples during the newborn period from their influence after breast-feeding is well established. Type A refers to the infant's difficulty in exhibiting the correct oral configuration, latching technique, and suckling pattern necessary to extract milk from the breast after exposure to an artificial nipple. Typically this phenomenon occurs when the artificial nipple is introduced before the successful establishment of breast-feeding. It is especially likely to occur when the artificial nipple results in more rapid or altered flow of fluid than is available from the breast.

The term should not be applied to situations in which a newborn infant displays a primary inability to suckle the breast effectively, without exposure to an artificial nipple, pacifier or adult's finger. The term should only apply to an infant who successfully has been offered an artificial nipple and subsequently has had difficulty breast-feeding.

Type B refers to the older infant who is proficient at breast-feeding and then refuses the bottle. This is actually "bottle refusal" instead of nipple confusion. It can also describe infants who turn to the bottle and then start to refuse the breast. This may actually be related to decreased maternal milk supply or lack of interest in nursing.

The notion that a single bottle is likely to result in breast-feeding failure runs contrary to experience. Many breast-fed infants receive one or more supplemental feedings by bottle the first week of life and go on to breast-feed exclusively. Cronenwett, et al, in a study of 121 breast-feeding couples highly motivated to nurse, found that single bottle use daily in the early weeks after birth had no significant impact on the duration of breast-feeding.

No data exist to document the incidence of nipple confusion, the possible mechanisms involved in its cause or specific maternal and infant factors that may predispose an infant to difficulty in breast-feeding after exposure to an artificial nipple.

The therapist should carefully investigate the following risk factors to get to the heart of the feeding problem. Easy labels such as "nipple confusion" do not promote diagnostic therapy and complex treatment programs that are often needed to help infants with these subtle, multi-factoral feeding problems.

Maternal factors that may lead to feeding problems include: variability in nipple size, flat, inverted, long nipples, abnormal breasts that are hypoplastic or asymmetrical, previous breast surgery that has severed milk ducts, delayed or absent lactogenesis, low milk supply, hyperlactation, maternal illness, maternal-infant separation and difficulty learning proper technique.

Infant factors include: prematurity <37 weeks and subsequent neurological/neuromuscular, physiological challenges to feeding related to prematurity, APGAR <5 at one minute or <7 at five minutes, SGA, LGA, IUGR, infant of a diabetic mother, hypoglycemia, multiple births, illness, neonatal hyperbilirubinemia especially requiring phototherapy, down syndrome, hypotonia, dysfunctional sucking, oral anatomical problems: high palate, cleft lip/palate, micrognathia (small jaw) or difficulty latching on to the sustain sucking.

Breastfeeding

Breastmilk is composed of fat, water, human growth factors, human immunoglobins, digestive enzymes and bioactive agents. It is designed to uniquely meet the needs of the growing infant. It contains host-resistant factors including active enzymes, living cells, immunoglobins, hormones, carrier proteins and non-specific factors that protect the infant's respiratory and gastrointestinal tract from invasion by bacteria, viruses and other pathogens.

Hormones associated with breastmilk include prolactin which makes the milk inside the cells and oxytocin which allows for let down of milk.

Recent studies have shown that breastfeeding for four months, exclusively, reduces the risks of childhood diabetes, Crohn's disease, and childhood cancers, especially acute leukemia. Prospective studies of infants exclusively breastfed for six months and at high risk for allergies, such as infantile eczema, infant-onset asthma, and rhinitis have shown a lower-than-predicted onset of symptoms during the first two years of life. (Lawrence)

The first three days after delivery the mother produces colostrum which is high in fat and calories. Colostrum is very beneficial to the NICU infant due to the high risk of necrotizing enterocolitis. Mothers are urged to express colostrum even if they do not wish to breastfeed so that it can be given to the baby as "medicine" for the gut. Usually after the third day true breastmilk is produced.

THE MECHANICS OF BREASTFEEDING

Breastfeeding is different from bottle in method and technique. With breast, the baby opens his mouth and the milk flows in and he closes his mouth to compress the breast and stop the flow of milk. With bottle, the baby closes his mouth around the nipple and compresses it; he builds negative pressure in the mouth and extracts fluid from the nipple. When the baby opens the mouth, the flow of milk stops.

ADVANTAGES OF BREASTFEEDING

- Decreased ear infections
- Decreased allergies to food and environmental agents
- Decreased episodes of diarrhea
- Decreased respiratory infections
- Decreased risk of diabetes and cancer
- Increased IQ
- Thicker gut wall
- Mother's immunities are passed to the infant

ADVANTAGES TO THE MOTHER

- Quicker return to pre-pregnancy weight
- Decreased risk of breast cancer
- Increased bonding with the infant

BREASTFEEDING TRENDS

Surprisingly, working mother's breastfeed more than stay-at-home mothers. The #1 reason mothers stop exclusively breastfeeding is the notion that there is an inadequate milk supply. Babies go through several growth spurts or "frequency feeding" periods and mothers may report; "All he wants to do is nurse." They feel they have an inadequate supply of milk when the fact is this is a normal stage that occurs at 2-3 weeks and again between 4-6 weeks of age. Mothers may feel they are not producing enough milk to meet the infant's nutritional needs. Milk supply is a direct result of adequate stimulation to the nipple to stimulate production of prolactin. Prolactin produces the milk. If the mother truly does have an inadequate supply of milk, she needs to feed the baby more frequently or pump to increase production. If she is ready to wean the baby, she needs to allow more time between feedings.

COMPLICATIONS

Many complications of breastfeeding can be solved with a few helpful hints. Sore nipples are usually as a result of poor or incorrect latch-on and problems with positioning. Once appropriate positioning is achieved the mother begins to feel relief from the pain. A mother can be reassured about her milk supply during "growth spurts" when an infant is feeding frequently by calculation of the number of wet diapers and bowel movements an infant has throughout the day.

Some difficulties require medical intervention such as clogged duct or mastitis. Clogged ducts can be treated with massage and placing the baby's chin or nose where the clog is to help it move and disappear and if clog does not move within 24-48 hours a physician should be notified. Mastitis is an infection in the breast. Symptoms include fever, chills, vomiting, red streaks and a shiny look to the breast tissue. It may be a staph infection if one breast is involved or strep if both are affected. Mastitis occurs very rapidly and antibiotics and medical intervention are needed as soon as possible. It is important (although painful) to keep nursing and keep milk flowing so an abscess does not form.

BREASTFEEDING THE SPECIAL NEEDS INFANT

Preemies

The mother is separated from her baby and the baby may be critically ill. Double pumping is helpful in maintaining and increasing the milk supply. To put a preemie to breast, the infant should be 34 weeks with a weight of 1300 grams. The baby should have good oral reflexes and a good suck-swallow-breathe sequence.

A smaller baby can be put to breast (only for stimulation of the milk supply) during K-Care. Be sure the mother knows the smaller baby is not expected to be able to breastfeed or she may feel she has failed.

Down Syndrome

Babies present with low tone, weak suck, and depressed reflexes, which can interfere with effective nursing. Positioning and supplemental nursing systems/nipple shields may be helpful.

Cleft Palate

The baby with a cleft palate imprints on the first method of feeding very quickly and may have difficulty transitioning from bottle to breast. The baby has difficulty creating a vacuum to hold the breast in the oral cavity. A supplemental nursing system may work for some infants.

The parents should be instructed in techniques to provide external support. Other feeding methods may need to be explored, such as using a Y-cut Dr. Brown Nipple and Bottle system, a cleft palate nurser or the Pigeon nipple and bottle.

BABY-FRIENDLY HOSPITALS

These hospitals create an environment, which supports women and their desire to breastfeed. The staff provides assistance and implements policies which safeguard the breastfeeding relationship. It is important to support the mother who is uncomfortable with breastfeeding. If the mother wishes to pump her milk and give it to the baby in a bottle, she is still breastfeeding by providing breast milk to her baby.

BENEFITS FOR PREMATURE INFANTS
1. Achieve full feedings more quickly by increasing tolerance.
2. Decrease site of infection.
3. Incidence of infection is lower for the baby who receives breastmilk because of the decrease in intestinal permeability.
4. Decreased risk of NEC secondary to protecting the gut wall from infection.
5. Breastmilk contains an anti-inflammatory property which promotes healing (regurgitation with less scarring) and also contains growth hormones).
6. Long term effects include protection against allergy and asthma, increase in visual acuity, increase in IQ, increase in retinal development (lipids in the milk assist in development), Omega 3 and Omega 6 contribute to growth of the nervous system. Omega 3 and 6 would have been passed to the infant during the third trimester had the baby been carried to term. It can be passed through the breastmilk, but is not present in formula.
7. Preterm milk is higher in fat than term milk.

Recommendations
for the Mother of a Premature Infant

- Use a hospital grade pump to elicit the amount of stimulation needed to increase prolactin levels.
- During the first two weeks after delivery it is recommended that the mother pump 8 to 10 times per day or to maximize milk supply pump 12 times per day.
- During the first two weeks the average milk yield to sustain growth is 350-400cc/day. By day ten the ideal milk volume is 750cc/day.
- Imagery can increase milk supply. The mother should use of a picture of the baby or an article of clothing to think about the baby while pumping. In some nurseries the mother is allowed to pump at bedside. Many mothers are anxious and fearful when away from their baby. The mother

is more relaxed at bedside because she can monitor her baby's status. Pumping during K-care is also an option that is proven to increase milk yield by 50%. The mother needs to associate let down with the baby, not the sound of the pump.

LACTOENGINEERING

Types of milk: Foremilk, Hindmilk, Hind-hind mild, and Composite Milk.

When the mother pumps for 15 to 20 minutes she produces composite milk, which is a combination of foremilk, hind milk and hind-hind milk. Lactoengineering measures the creamatocrit of the milk. The milk is fractionated and a percentage of volume (which is cream) is obtained. Pumping to collect hind milk can increase calories by 300%. When hind-hind milk is used 65% of the milk calories come from fat. This rich milk can greatly increase the infant's weight gain.

KANGAROO CARE

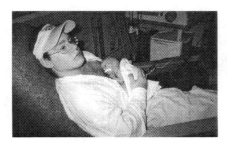

Skin-to-skin contact provided during Kangaroo Care allows an infant to maintain their body temperature while stabilizing the infant's heart and respiratory rates.

▲ *Dad and baby in KCare* ▲

While doing kangaroo care the infant is placed against the bare chest of either parent. Research has shown that this provides the baby with physiological stability by stabilizing the heart and respiratory rate and body temperature. EEG patterns show longer, uninterrupted periods of deep sleep, which helps in secreting growth hormones. Metabolic activity in the breasts keeps the infant warmer with a more consistent temperature than a warming bed. Fathers can do K-care but the infant needs temperature monitoring.

Pacifiers

There is no research that shows using a pacifier with a preterm infant interferes with breastfeeding. Pacifiers are actually encouraged during gavage feedings and their use results in better GI transit time, an increase in fat breakdown and better weight gain. The infant also associates a feeling of fullness with oral stimulation. Pacifiers can calm an infant that results in better state and organization and as a result less energy expenditure.

CHAPTER SEVEN

▲

Treatment Programs

T his chapter is designed to serve as a quick reference guide for the busy therapist. Please check our references for additional resources for treatment. We have combined the work and research of many different authors from many disciplines to create a comprehensive listing of treatment ideas.

Chat Time: Specific Infant Treatment Strategies

TTREATMENT RESOURCES

Feeding and Swallowing Disorders in Infancy by Wolf and Glass, *Childhood Feeding Disorder: Biobehavioral Assessment and Intervention* by Kedesky and Budd and *Prefeeding Skills* by Suzanne Evans Morris are excellent resources for treatment strategies. We encourage a combination approach of Wolf and Glass, Joan Arvedson, Rona Alexander, Suzanne Evans Morris, Catherine Shaker and Marjorie Meyer Palmer's strategies, but also that the therapist develop their intervention programs based on the needs of the child.

Treatment strategies are simply suggestions about what might work or has worked for some children. Evaluate thoroughly and pull ideas from the other professionals involved in the child's care into your program. Oral sensory-motor treatment strategies, with age appropriate mouthing programs, compliment oral motor feeding therapy and should be explored by the therapist.

Occupational therapists can also help the speech pathologist develop multi-sensory treatment programs to improve the effectiveness of the feeding program. Dietitian's input is vital to the treatment. Children with multiple health issues will need the support of home-health nursing and medical personnel and treatment must bring all of these professionals together for a positive outcome to intervention.

TRAINING

It is the therapist's responsibility to train with experienced therapists and to develop their skills and knowledge base prior to taking on these challenging patients. There is no cookbook for therapy with neonatal infants or older graduates/young children. The main point is to treat the whole body to treat feeding. Combinations of any or all of the following may be used in treating an infant. Daily re-assessment of the infant is part of your treatment program. Always know why you are in the unit or in treatment and what your goals are for each session. This will keep you focused and help you explain your program to nurses and physicians, as well as family members.

PARENTS

Train parents/caregivers as primary feeders. The parent should be the one who feeds his or her child better than anyone else. Don't take that away from a parent. Work to help them help their child, then every feeding can be therapeutic instead of just the ones conducted by the therapist. Some families require a great deal of special handling, instruction and patience. Take the time to treat the entire family to help the child and to give your intervention program the greatest chance of success.

NIPPLE CHOICE

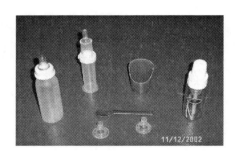

These feeding devices are just a few of the tools used to help build strength and stability in the oral musculature while feeding. When choosing an appropriate tool for feeding you must know the impact to the oral, pharyngeal, and esophageal stages of the swallow.

▲ *Bottles, Nipples, Spoons* ▲

Using the appropriate nipple to feed a preemie or newborn is a critical part of your treatment protocol. Nipples vary greatly in quality. Gerber silicone slow or medium flow and the Dr. Brown Bottles with Level I or II nipples are very good choices for most NICU graduates. We recommend these products because they facilitate the development of tongue grooving and activate the cheeks and the flow rate is appropriate for most infants who fed well on the yellow nipple. We do not recommend that an infant be sent home on the red preemie nipple. Refer to the nipple comparison chart in Chapter 11 for detailed information.

ENDURANCE PROBLEMS

Fatigue and endurance issues are common in babies with BPD, cardiac problems, RDS, motor problems and hypersensitivity (babies who sleep as a way of tuning out the overstimulating environment). The therapist needs to find a way to feed the baby with as little physical effort as possible. The baby must have adequate rest between feedings. You may recommend one or all of the following:

- Reduce environmental stimulation so the baby is focused only on feeding and can rest adequately between feedings.
- Feed with at least three hours recovery time after a feeding on a demand schedule when appropriate.
- If you feed ad lib remember to limit nippling time to 20-30 minutes, don't let the family fall into a grazing pattern. Many parents misinterpret crying/fussiness as hunger and use the bottle for calming. Teach alternative calming strategies or refer to occupational therapy.
- Increase calories in the formula or have the mother pump hind milk (lactoengineering) so the baby does not have to take as much formula.

- Support and position the baby by swaddling well (but with an unrestricted chest and abdomen) and provide jaw and cheek support if necessary. Chin support stabilizes the mandible and allows the cheek muscles to function more efficiently and with less effort.
- Evaluate oxygen saturation levels. Hypoxemia could be occurring resulting in lethargy and drowsiness. Babies with respiratory problems may need supplemental oxygen during feedings.
- Make sure the baby's ribcage is slightly extended with an open chest and abdomen for optimal respiratory and digestive function.
- Discuss the infant's physical condition with the nurse or physician to determine if there is a less obvious cause for the fatigue (low hematocrit, etc.).

POOR SUCK.

Sucking is not consistently achieved until the infant reaches 37 weeks post-conceptional age. Premature infants have difficulty developing stability in the tongue and jaw. The infant lacks the brown fat layer that comes in closer to term. This layer gives the baby stability through the body and fat pads on the cheeks. The fat pads provide stability and allow the tongue/lips to work optimally. The baby also may exhibit poor muscle control in the neck; trunk and pelvis, which may impact, jaw stability. Older babies may also have poor tone, inactive cheek musculature and poor lip seal.

- Develop an oral exercise program that alerts and prepares the baby for nippling attempts. This can include stimulation or deep pressure to the palate, gum ridge and lips/tongue.
- Stimulate the root reflex frequently providing firm pressure touch to the cheek and move gently in toward the mouth, then stroke down the center of the lower lip (preemies). The goal is to encourage the baby to initiate the sucking pattern. This allows for optimal learning of this skill and usually the tongue drops into the appropriate position for nippling.
- Provide a therapeutic pacifier (Soothie or Wee-Soothie) for non-nutritive sucking and provide slight traction as the baby is sucking the pacifier to work the musculature (repeat 2-3 times, three or four times per day).
- Support under the chin, on the bone, and to the cheeks (lightly) if needed to encourage activation and provide stability to the structures. Provide cheek support and then release periodically during the feeding to see if the muscle is activated. Do not put pressure on the musculature under the jaw as you can inhibit movement of the floor muscles of the tongue and compromise the swallow.
- Slow-medium flow nipple.
- Downward pressure on the tongue with the nipple can encourage good tongue grooving if it is diminished or absent.
- With preemies, you are looking for suck/pauses of equal duration, do not encourage the baby to suck again during their natural breathing pauses as this can lead to a significant desaturation. If the pause is excessively long, slight rolling or upward pressure with the nipple on the hard palate can stimulate sucking.
- Monitor the swallow carefully; poor suck and poor oral/pharyngeal control place the baby at significant risk for premature spillage into the

Evaluation and Treatment of Pediatric Feeding Disorders: From NICU to Childhood

pharynx and microaspiration. Daily reassessment via cervical auscultation is strongly recommended.

- Oral exploration of toys/teethers in the older child paired with very small therapeutic tastes to regain or improve rhythmical sucking patterns.

POOR COORDINATION OF THE SUCK-SWALLOW-BREATHE SEQUENCE

Read the infant's cues to observe stress signals (color change, breathing rate changes, chin tugging, audible swallows, oral spillage, multiple swallows and coughing/choking) while nippling. Imposed breaks (tip bottle down, do not remove the bottle from the mouth over and over) are needed until the baby can coordinate the S/S/B sequence. Breaks decrease fatigue, pace energy expenditure, provide time to reorganize breathing, promote deep breathing, provide time to clear the mouth or throat and slow the infant down when he is gulping. Try some of the following techniques:

- Swaddle the baby to reduce sensation to the rest of the body and focus on the mouth, as well as providing midline stability. For unrestricted respiration, keep the chest open and loosen the diaper if needed.
- Modified upright sidelying positioning may be effective as milk will collect briefly in the buccal area and this mimics breastfeeding positioning.
- Optimal positioning of the body for efficient breathing, support and digestion, consult occupational therapist if needed.
- If coordination is very poor, you may have to give the baby single bolus swallows via the Hazelbaker Finger Feeder or syringe and pacifier to provide bolus formulation practice. Swallow study (MBS/VFSS/FEES) may be needed.
- Size of the bolus can have a significant effect on breathing and swallowing, so limit the size by using a slow or medium flow nipple (standard Ross yellow for inpatients, Gerber slow or medium flow, Dr. Brown Bottle with Level II nipple for a market brand product).
- May need thickened feedings (we suggest using blenderized rice cereal or oatmeal) to avoid slit nipples or regular cereal can be used with the Dr. Brown Bottle and Y-cut nipple. Never cut or slit a nipple. It is very difficult to thicken breastmilk and a slow flow nipple may be the best option for expressed feedings. At the breast, the mother may need to pump prior to putting the baby to breast to reduce flow rate and initial bursts of breastmilk. Appropriate positioning techniques at breast can also protect the baby from rapid let down. Monitor via cervical auscultation.
- Continue to impose breaks and then wait and see if the baby pauses on his/her own.
- Some babies respond to light rocking of the bottle to teach rhythm.
- Oral motor stimulation to improve suck/swallow.
- With older children, sucking still occurs on the bottle or cup.

Remember, Thick-It may cause increased constipation in some children and taste sensitive children may refuse it completely. See alternatives to Thick-It in the cup drinking guidelines. Make sure positioning is perfect, look out for cervical hyperextension and give small sips as tolerated. Teach children to "drink and stop." Some children with cerebral palsy have a difficult time regulating their intake of liquids and will not pause adequately to breathe.

ORAL-FACIAL HYPERSENSITIVITY/ EARLY FEEDING AVERSION

For optimal communication with medical staff/insurance providers, be sure to label medical disorders that impact feeding appropriately and indicate that feeding aversion is a *consequence* of the specific problem. The baby has often experienced unpleasant and painful procedures as part of the medical care to save his life and he has been denied the normal stimulation to the face due to his prematurity and inability to nipple feed regularly. Techniques to reduce aversion/hypersensitivity include:

- Try to reduce negative medical procedures in the course of treatment. An indwelling silastic feeding tube may be less aversive than changing the nasogastric tube every few days; however; this varies baby to baby. Urge nursing staff to use as little tape on the face as possible.
- Offer a pacifier during tube feedings or Kangaroo Care if possible.
- Graded input working from the arms up to the face with firm pressure massage. Stop at any hint of discomfort or aversive response. Work slowly. Most babies respond to firm pressure on the face instead of stroking until they can handle more sensory input.
- Provide positive oral experiences and teach these techniques to caregivers. Some infants prefer deep pressure touch in a press and release pattern, others respond to very gradual, deep stroking of the cheeks in toward the lips.
- Gradually introduce the pacifier when infant demonstrates readiness. Non-nutritive suck accelerates maturation of the sucking response, helps the baby switch to oral feedings faster, improves oxygen saturation levels, calms and pacifies the baby, improves gastrointestinal function, helps with weight gain, improves muscle tone and coordination of the suck/swallow/breathe sequence and contributes to earlier discharge dates.
- When the infant can accept the pacifier, work toward tolerance of liquid by dipping the pacifier in formula or breastmilk or using the Hazelbaker Finger Feeder or syringe and pacifier for tastes. Work up from single bolus swallows to successive swallows to small feedings. If the infant demonstrates signs of swallow difficulty, request a modified barium swallow study.
- Chilled formula works well for some infants. Be sure to clear use of thermal stimulation with the physician.
- Appropriate flow rate and type of nipple is critical to the treatment program.
- Infant may need assessment and treatment by occupational therapist.

Chat Time: Child Friendly Treatment Programs

ORAL MOTOR THERAPY IS MORE THAN THE NUK BRUSH

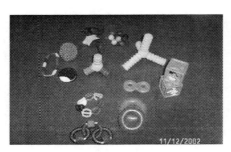

▲ *Teethers* ▲

Oral play with teethers and toys are encouraged for all children; these tools are therapeutic for those who experience texture or spoon aversions. Teethers provide a variety of textures to teach the child about his mouth and to desensitize the gag reflex in a non-threatening manner. Dipping a teether is also an excellent way to introduce a new taste of pureed food.

Oral-motor exercise programs need to be fun and functional. We use the Nuk brush in our treatment sessions; but there are so many wonderful alternatives out there that should be explored. We primarily use the Nuk as a spoon for children who don't like texture or for specific treatment plans. We dip the Nuk in smooth foods and watch where the child puts the brush in his own mouth. We also use the other Nuk brushes in the package of three with the soft brush and brush with the small ridges.

There are a wide variety of appropriate mouthing toys for infants and children of all ages. Get plastic containers or zip lock bags to hold mouthing toys for your patients and be creative. Always clean your mouthing toys thoroughly.

Use a mirror in treatment to give the child additional input. Puppets that swallow (available from New Visions) or sock puppets that you make in treatment are great for your oral exercise programs. We use only latex free gloves during our sessions; powdered latex gloves should not be used during oral motor treatment.

A FEW EXAMPLES OF THE TRIED AND TRUE

Some children will be able to tolerate these activities and others due to their sensory needs will not. Adjust these ideas as needed or do them on yourself initially to introduce the activity and so the child can learn from observation. Give the child only the input they can tolerate at each stage of treatment.

Don't ever force oral input on children, they have the right to refuse treatment like any other patient. An oral exercise program can take weeks or months to fully implement the plan. Oral exercises are a "conversation", you touch a child's face and they respond and you adjust your input dependent on the response given. This back and forth communication should continue with all of your patients, no matter what the age.

Increased respiratory and heart rate signal discomfort with some children, maintain contact, but roll your fingers/hand(s) back slowly while maintaining deep pressure. Wait and observe the child. If the child is breathing easier and tolerating the input, maintain that position and ever so slowly progress forward again. Many times this is so slow your hands don't even look like they are moving. Pressure must be adequate and many therapists underestimate this need.

Treatment Programs

If the child turns away or shows continued distress, he is telling you something; start treatment away from the face at the hands or shoulders or again, adjust the pressure level. Give the child time and the type of input he can tolerate. Pressure level/rate of movement must be appropriate.

Consult with occupational therapy to make sure your treatment plan meets the child's needs. Follow these activities with a functional activity, such as, bottle/cup drinking or a small snack.

Lip Exercises

Exercises for lip closure and activation should be fun and functional. We use a maroon spoon or flavored tongue depressor and put pixie stix powder or cake frosting only on the tip and have a competition to see who can get it all off in one attempt by squeezing the lips tightly on the spoon or tongue depressor.

Have the child hold the tongue depressor in the mouth and pretend it is a diving board. The therapist can "walk" on the tongue depressor with two fingers and "jump" on the end. We also use small toys to "walk the plank" in our treatment sessions. Use make-up brushes or soft paintbrushes and face paint, coat the lips with pudding and make kiss imprints on paper.

Thera-band (use latex free) is great to use to give deep input to the upper and lower lip, pull it tightly and "outline" the lips above and below with deep pressure input. Be creative and have fun, the possibilities are endless.

Cheeks

Are the cheeks too tight or too loose? Give the right input dependent on what you want to accomplish. Make funny faces in a mirror, have the child pull the cheeks in and make "fish faces" and hold it or give deep input with your hands while you sing songs or play music, such as Disney's "Under the Sea."

The kids will enjoy it and be motivated to hold the posture much longer this way than in a dry oral exercise drill. Massage and give deep input to the face paired with songs or finger plays. We tell the kids their cheeks "fell off" and find them in our pockets and in a firm press touch "put their cheeks back on." Put them in the wrong place too, press under the lower lip and have the child tell you if you put their cheek back in the right place. This is a good sensory activity and they laugh and enjoy treatment.

Have the child puff air in the cheeks and squish it out by pushing both hands into the musculature. Use a Nuk brush covered by an Infa-dent and dipped in a carbonated beverage to give input to the inner cheeks. Function of the inner cheek is very important to saliva management and effective feeding. Make the child aware of the inner cheek by chilling the brush and rolling it or tapping it down the musculature.

Pretend the cheeks are asleep and you have to wake them up. Use gloved index and middle fingers and place on outside on the cheek and one inside to shake or stretch the muscle. Be cautious with children who have a tonic bite reflex. Watch those fingers!

Tongue

Oh the possibilities! Tell stories with and provide sound effects with tongue pops and clicks; put cotton candy in different areas on the lips and see if the child can use the tongue to find it; for lateralization hold gummy worms or goldfish crackers on dental floss by the corner of the mouth and have the child try to make contact with the tongue. Sings songs with "la, la, la" and see if the tongue is "awake" to sing.

If the child is not moving the tongue well, use the Nuk or a teether and "knock" on the teeth to see if the tongue is awake. Pop Rocks can also be used to wake up the tongue. Tongue walk with the Nuk or use a vibrating teether toy (not appropriate for a child with a history of seizure disorder) to provide input to the tongue. Cover your face with a towel or blanket and make a funny face, lower the cover and see if the child can imitate your facial expression and posture. Their timing and imitation should improve over time. Have fun with your patients, siblings are great to work with during these activities as well and this is a great way to get carry-over for your program.

Jaw

Biting toys are great for playing "puppy dog." Practice big bites (big dog) vs little bites (little dog) and let the child learn the difference. Use music and bite hard when the music is loud and bite soft when the volume is reduced. Bite on frozen washcloths, hard licorice sticks, vibrating star teethers and then give deep input to the center of each tooth with the tip of the Nuk brush. Let the child feel this input down through the jaw.

Give input across the mandible by tapping or deep pressure and use the mirror to show the child where their jawbone is located. Face-paint the jaw or make shaving cream or Cool Whip beards by covering the mandible. Play "garage" and have the garage door (jaw or teeth) open when the child opens the mouth and see if the car (tongue) is inside.

Drooling Management

Try to increase awareness of a dry vs. a wet chin. Use a washcloth to dry the chin or the children can wear a wristband to wipe the face themselves; they just need to learn to feel the difference. Again, use the mirror so they can see that they are drooling (be careful not to hurt their feelings, don't embarrass them in front of other children) and use positive, fun language to tell them "uh-oh, the water is on, let's turn it off" as a swallow cue.

Make sure the chin is dry, assist with jaw closure and occasionally give the lightest stroke down the larynx if needed. Do this on yourself first to model for the child and also to feel that only the lightest input is needed. *Do not do this often; this can become very aversive to a child.* A small tap to the chin can become the swallow cue instead of the stroke to the larynx. Wait for a swallow.

Fish face games can also be used during secretion management sessions to improve lip closure and to draw the cheeks in toward the tongue to assist with an efficient swallow. Use the puppet and model a "gulp" sound as the "water" is pushed down to the tummy. Use language a child understands and can relate to and give him/her time; secretion management is very challenging.

Inappropriate positioning, fatigue, low tone in the oral facial region, reflux and poor nutrition can contribute to problems with secretion management. There are medications that reduce drooling by thickening saliva, however, there are side effects and the child may not be able to safely clear thickened secretions. Team evaluation and treatment is needed.

CHAPTER EIGHT

▲

Evaluation and Treatment of Feeding Aversion

"Behavioral therapy for feeding disorders has been comprehensively reviewed. A combination of social praise and a program that makes the consumption of preferred foods contingent on eating non-preferred foods is often successful in modifying eating behaviors. Contingency strategies, "shaping" by rewarding successive approximation of targeted behaviors, "positive reinforcement" by rewarding a child with praise or access to favored toys, and "ignoring" or inattention when the child engages in inappropriate behaviors are all used to modify feeding behaviors. Successful implementation of these management approaches usually requires a structured inpatient management program with frequent outpatient follow-up care. Children with physiological or anatomic disorders often can improve feeding skills with modification of nipple type, feeding utensils, or food consistency. Changes in position during feeding and learning specific maneuvers to avoid aspiration during feeds also may decrease the risk of aspiration."
--Rudolph C: Feeding Disorders in Infants and Children.
Journal of Pediatrics 1994; 125:S116-24.

Red Flags for Future Feeding Difficulties or Feeding Aversion

- Oral-motor dysfunction
- Dysphagia
- MH of diagnoses that lead to feeding disruption (i.e. BPD, RDS, cardiac problems, neurological impairment, GERD, etc.)
- History of prolonged intubation or suctioning (negative oral experiences)
- Supplemental tube feedings (can reduce sensation of hunger)
- Failure to match diet to developmental age
- Poor meal scheduling
- Poor/inappropriate parental feeding strategies

Feeding aversion can be defined as self-restriction of type, texture or amount of food available to a child. A feeding aversion can range from mild to severe in nature.

A mild aversion refers to children who may be classified as "picky eaters." Generally, a mild feeding aversion does not effect a child's development or overall health. However, a severe feeding aversion refers to an extreme self-restriction of intake, which leads to significant developmental, social and health problems. A severe feeding aversion left untreated can lead to failure to thrive. (Kedesdy and Budd)

Overview of the Team Approach

To adequately treat an individual with a feeding aversion a team approach of multiple professionals may be necessary. A multidisciplinary team is developed based on the child's individual needs and may include the following members the primary care physician, pediatric gastroenterologist, psychologist, otolaryngologist, dietitian, nursing service, speech-language pathologist, occupational therapist, physical therapist, lactation consultant, social work service and child-life specialist.

Evaluation will begin with a complete physical examination to determine if there are underlying medical issues impacting feeding. An oral-motor and swallowing evaluation will be completed to rule out dysphagia. Bonding and the interaction between the child and parent will be assessed to see if more successful interaction can occur. Positioning will be assessed and adaptive equipment may be ordered. The child may be treated initially as an outpatient or in certain cases admitted to the hospital for intensive therapy and behavioral intervention to improve intake.

Treatment may be on an inpatient or outpatient basis and may include setting a schedule of three meals, three snacks per day. The team will analyze patterns of food and liquid intake to see if there is a grazing pattern that is decreasing the child's appetite. Meals may be limited to 30 to 45 minutes and snacks to 10 to 20. Generally meals are 20 to 30 minutes and snacks are 10 to 15 minutes, however, some children require additional time. The program should fit the needs of the child.

Mealtime behaviors will be analyzed to determine the scope of the feeding problem and an initial program will be developed to increase positive behaviors and eliminate negatives. Parent/caregiver education will be provided by all team members via videotaped meals, direct instruction, and team meetings with the family to adjust the treatment program.

Treatment Guidelines: "The Rules"

THE EVALUATION PROCESS

Generally speaking, there are negotiable and non-negotiable rules for treatment of feeding disorders:

- All children should have a thorough oral motor/feeding/swallowing assessment and modified barium swallow studies should be completed on any child that shows symptoms of swallow dysfunction.
- A very thorough medical and feeding history must be taken to determine what is behavioral and what is physical, emotional and environmental. This requires assessment from a feeding team. Provide treatment for any underlying physical problem (reflux, constipation, etc.).
- Determine which foods are safe for the child and provide balanced choices of a variety of flavors. You are gathering information to see what food types/tastes/temperatures/consistencies are tolerated or accepted. Look carefully at rejected foods and look for patterns in taste/texture/temperature, this will help you develop your feeding program.

- Get growth records and plot the child's height, weight and head circumference growth patterns. The dietitian should analyze the child's feeding history and growth pattern to set goals for treatment. Some children will require supplemental feedings prior to implementation of a behavioral feeding program.

THE FEEDING ENVIRONMENT

Following assessment, set up a positive mealtime environment, determine what motivates the child and have a variety of reinforcers to reward positive feeding behaviors. Have a clear vision of behaviors that should be extinguished.

Not all behaviors interfere with successful mealtime experiences or reduce/prevent adequate intake. Focus on what must change for the child to eat well enough to meet his nutritional needs. These are the core behaviors to address in the beginning of the treatment program.

THE BEHAVIORAL PLAN

There should be an established, consistent plan regarding management of behaviors from the language used (scripts) to the amount and type of attention given to the child.

- The environment should be carefully controlled in regard to distraction, television and the people present in the room during therapeutic meals.
- Take time to educate the family to help them understand and feel comfortable with treatment techniques eliminate negative behaviors; this is key to the success of the program.
- Teach the parent/all caregivers to follow the program exactly. Videotape is a very powerful teaching tool. Don't miss feeders at school, daycare and extended family.
- Offer the child choices of two foods or food and drink. Let the child feel in control of the meal. Praise all positive behavior.
- Make sure you have set the child up to succeed and don't give them a large portion of food or all new foods. Success at first may be picking up a piece of food, tasting by licking a new food one time or no tantrums at a meal.
- Do not push a good feeding too far; know when to quit. This is punishing the child for a good meal.
- Stay within the scheduled mealtimes. Sometimes, new foods or transitional foods are only offered at snacks during a shortened less pressured meal.
- Eat with the child whenever possible. You want to set up a normal meal environment. Ignore crying, gagging (if not a sign of oral motor dysfunction or swallowing disorder), dropping food, throwing food and other behaviors that you wish to extinguish. Gradually work the parent/caregivers into the meal as primary feeder.

THE FEEDING SCHEDULE

- The schedule is three meals, two-three snacks a day.
- Duration of meals should be thirty-minute meals and fifteen-minute snacks. This is maximum time at the table; *it does not mean the child has to eat for thirty minutes.*
- No grazing (nibbling food or sipping liquids) is allowed between scheduled meals and snacks. The child can have water in a cup or bottle between scheduled intake, but no milk, juice, tea, soda. Milk is the only liquid allowed at meals and snacks. Children who are allergic to milk can have soymilk or in some cases NuBasics juice.
- The child cannot carry or have easy access to the cup or bottle or take any other type of food (candy, cookies, and crackers) except at meal or snack time. We want to use appetite to our advantage and children do not eat past the full point. Children have different hunger patterns than adults and must be treated by people experienced with pediatrics.
- Manipulation of food intake to stimulate appetite should be completed with the direction of a physician and dietitian. This in no way means, "He will eat when he is hungry enough." That method of treatment does not work!

THE RIGHT FOODS AT THE RIGHT TIME

- Gather information from the family listing all liquids/foods in the child's repertoire.
- Classify into categories of favorite foods, likes/dislikes and foods that are difficult to eat or cause gagging/choking problems.
- Have the family provide the team with three-day food logs to determine when the child is eating or drinking, what amounts are consumed and to assess caloric needs for optimal nutrition.
- Talk to the family and see what foods they normally prepare at mealtime. Take into consideration their lifestyle. Do they eat out frequently? Write your program to match their lifestyle.
- Add new foods that are similar to ones you have had success with.
- Provide the child with comfort foods that they are used to eating and a few tastes of new or transitional foods.
- Most children do not take caloric supplements (Nutren Jr. or Pediasure, Kindercal) during this phase of treatment.
- Find ways to modify the foods they are currently preparing for optimal success. Pediatric dietitians are very helpful in assisting the therapist in development of these programs and should be consulted. Request an order from the treating physician for a dietitian to evaluate the child. If you are providing home based services, call local hospitals and see if you can discuss treatment ideas/ schedule a session with a dietitian. The dietitian may also be able to be present at an office visit with the physician and help develop a food program with the family.

What Type of Aversion?
Mild vs. Extreme Selectivity: Typical Features
(Kedesky and Budd)

Kedesky and Budd's *Degree of Self-Restriction Scale* can be used in your evaluations to justify feeding therapy or to analyze features of the feeding disorder. Include descriptions of these areas of feeding in your report and take these findings into account when developing your treatment program.

MILD SELECTIVITY

The child may have strong preferences within food groups (eats chicken and pork and refuses beef), may refuse all members of a single food group, and may have strong flavor preferences.

EXTREME SELECTIVITY

The child may frequently reject all members of several food groups (may consume milk and peanut butter sandwiches exclusively) and may refuse any unsweetened food.

TEXTURE

Mild cases may prefer liquids or have some difficulty making the transition to advanced textures. Extreme cases may chronically resist developmentally appropriate textures and may have exclusive preference for single texture (liquid or pureed).

VOLUME

Mild cases meal portion size is frequently small, caloric intake may be highly variable but is satisfactory over time. Extreme cases may refuse to eat entirely (sustained by tube feeding) and caloric intake often suboptimal over time.

ASSOCIATED PROBLEMS

Mild cases present with recurrent mealtime struggles. Significant child/caregiver distress and strong emotional (phobic) reactions to the introduction of novel foods characterize extreme cases.

PERSISTENCE/RESPONSE TO INTERVENTION

Mild cases often are developmentally correlated; feeding problems are managed with parent guidance or short-term professional intervention. Extreme cases are usually chronic, resistant to brief interventions and require intensive, sustained, professional intervention.

CONSEQUENCES

Mild cases present no health or developmental consequences and there are limited social consequences. Extreme cases are high risk for health problems, sub-optimal nutrition, increased vulnerability to infection, poor growth, bone growth issues, significant developmental consequences (limited opportunity to practice oral-motor skills) and significant social consequences (unable to eat with family or peers).

Setting the Tone:
Environmental Intervention for Feeding Disorders
(Kedesky and Budd)

These environmental interventions are quick and easy techniques to add to your treatment program. Discuss the need for intervention in these areas with the parents/caregivers.

MEAL CHARACTERISTICS

Offer a developmentally appropriate menu and repeatedly offer a new or less preferred food as part of the meal. Children's tastes are changing and they may accept a new food once they have seen it on their plates several times. Make the meals colorful and attractive to the eye.

SCHEDULE OF INTAKE

Alter frequency of meals to promote appetite and limit length of meal to 10-20 minute snacks and 30-minute meals, depending on the child's cooperation. This is done to work toward the goal of internal motivation to eat by establishing appropriate hunger patterns.

SETTING CHARACTERISTICS

Reduce environmental distracters (television, toys, there are, however exceptions to this rule) and seat child in supported position for meals. The family should sit down and eat together.

INTERACTIONS

Attend and respond to child's hunger and satiety cues, provide pleasant social attention when child is cooperative and totally ignore when the child is disruptive or resistant. The child should not be the main focus of attention during meals. This is a family time and the child needs to learn that meals do not revolve around him.

OTHER INTERVENTIONS

Examples of these types of interventions include offering a pacifier for non-nutritive sucking during non-oral feedings and providing adaptive eating utensils to facilitate independent feeding skills.

Strategies to Increase Texture in Foods

Some infants and young children with feeding or texture aversion have difficulty transitioning from pureed consistencies to lumpier foods. The following guidelines are strategies to successfully make the transition:

- Begin with the consistency that the child will accept. For example, stage 2 baby food bananas.
- Using a baby food grinder, food processor, or blender, puree a real banana.
- Mix ¾ baby food with ¼ real banana; increase the ratio of the real banana and wean the baby food as the child tolerates the texture and taste of the table food.

As the child tolerates the transition from baby food to real food items, begin to increase the texture from smooth to lumpy:

- Use a Nuk brush (if tolerated), pacifier or textured teether as a spoon to administer the pureed food. The Nuk brush or toy adds a degree of texture as the child accepts the bite.
- Use finely crushed crackers, pretzels, and vanilla wafer cookies into the pureed food. Increase the amount that is added or size of the pieces as the child tolerates.
- Keeping tastes the same, add small pieces of the real food to the pureed mixture. For example place small pieces of a banana into a pureed banana mixture. Increase the size of the pieces as the child tolerates.

The Right Food at the Right Time: Food Chaining
(Fraker and Walbert)

"Chaining" refers to taking accepted foods/liquids in the repertoire and modifying or linking them to other specifically selected foods/liquids. This is an excellent way to expand a child's food repertoire and is especially effective with the child with severely restricted food choices. This technique can also work very well with children who have autistic spectrum disorder. We developed this treatment strategy based on the belief that we all have categories of preferred tastes/texture/temperature of food. We all eat foods we like and this technique helps find patterns in the preferred foods, as well as rejected food lists.

Chaining foods by flavor, texture and consistency is a good idea for all feeding patients. Food chains may be developed for children with mild to severe aversions; sensory based food refusals or behavioral food refusals. Food chains are customized for each patient and can be simple or extremely complex. Several examples of food chains developed for children are included in this chapter to help explain this treatment strategy. The first case involved a child with a severely restricted food repertoire; her name is Holly.

CASE EXAMPLE: HOLLY

History

Holly was a three-year-old child who demonstrated severe food selectivity from age 6 months. The pediatric gastroenterologist, behavioral psychologist, dietitian, speech and occupational therapist evaluated this patient and determined that she would be an excellent candidate for a food-chaining program. The speech pathologist/feeding specialist and dietitian developed Holly's food chains. Holly had a very restricted diet and rejected new foods by sight. The nine-food/drink items listed (see food chain chart) were the only table foods she had ever accepted. She was not consistently eating all of the foods listed but had demonstrated some degree of past success with them.

At the time of the initial consultation, Holly's diet consisted of only strawberry-kiwi juice and crackers and she would occasionally eat Burger King French fries. Holly was started on caloric supplements (NuBasics Juice) for several weeks prior to starting the feeding program. We made this recommendation to improve weight and general health to prepare for the treatment program. When treatment began, caloric supplements were discontinued to let Holly feel hungry at meal and snack times.

Holly's medical history was significant for mild prematurity. She was born at 35 weeks gestation and had asthma and frequent illnesses. Evaluation by the pediatric gastroenterologist did not reveal any underlying reason for Holly's aversion. Evaluation of the swallow was normal. Holly had also been evaluated by an occupational therapist in the past but treatment was not successful. Holly had severe anxiety issues around new people and would not allow the occupational therapist to interact with her in treatment. Our occupational therapist re-evaluated Holly and assisted the team in development of a sensory-based treatment program as well as providing a home program to her family. The behavior psychologist was consulted to evaluate Holly's cognitive, social and emotional development, analyze her behaviors and counsel her parents in techniques to deal with her strong fear of new people and situations.

Treatment

Due to Holly's reluctance to participate in sessions with team members, meals were videotaped at home and shared with our feeding team for analysis of mealtime behaviors. Holly presented with signs of tactile hypersensitivity on her hands, but did not respond aversely to food on her face. She appeared to have intra-oral hyposensitivity and preferred foods that were crunchy, salty or chewy. Food logs were analyzed and a detailed feeding history was reported by the dietitian to team members. Holly presented with a grazing pattern of intake, she drank juice from her cup throughout the day and nibbled on crackers from a large bowl filled daily by her family. Her parents felt if she was eating something they felt less anxious and they believed the constant supply of food was the best way to deal with her feeding problem. In interviews with her parents it was revealed that Holly's food selectivity began with baby food. She would accept only one type of baby food and rejected all others. At age two she ate pancakes at each meal for several months and then rejected them completely. This pattern was repeated over and over as Holly would eat large amounts of one preferred food and then refuse it without warning. Holly did not appear to enjoy eating and she demonstrated tantrum behaviors when called to the table and cried/protested throughout the entire meal. Holly's mother was extremely stressed by her daughter's feeding behaviors and she was very concerned about her nutritional status.

Initial therapy goals addressed shaping mealtime behaviors and gradually expanding food repertoire. Holly rejected new foods on sight and would scream and cry when a new food was placed on her plate. When she was angry, Holly had a history of "hunger strike" behaviors and would often go two or three days without eating. Due to her parent's extreme anxiety about the possibility of additional food strike behaviors, foods were initially introduced during snack times only. New foods were placed in a bowl beside her plate in the beginning days of treatment and gradually introduced to her plate. Negative behaviors resulted in Holly being removed from the table. The behavior program focused on eliminating tantrums/negative behaviors at the table. These behaviors would simply not be tolerated. Holly was placed in her chair for meals and if she acted out, her parent attempted once more to bring her to the table. If she still refused or tantrumed, she was removed from the dining area and her meal was over until the next scheduled meal or snack. She was only offered water until the next scheduled meal or snack. Her parents were instructed to go into "robot mode" and totally ignore her outbursts, no matter how extreme. Crying would not hurt her, poor eating could. The team cautioned the family that all behaviors would escalate in the beginning phase of treatment, but they were also cautioned that if they gave in to her behaviors even one time they would increase the chances of the behavior occurring again by 300%. The team provided constant support to Holly's parents during this intensive phase of treatment. Holly's mother reported daily feeding behaviors via voice mail to the speech pathologist/feeding specialist and was contacted by team members on a daily basis to provide encouragement and direction.

Results

Consistent behavioral strategies, peer modeling, scheduled meals and snacks, appetite enhancing activities and a monthly food-chaining schedule were provided to the family. Holly's meals and snacks were scheduled and she no longer had a cup of juice to carry around all day. The team had a goal of developing internal motivation to eat. Holly needed to make good choices. When food was offered, she needed to learn that the expectation was for her to eat at that time. Holly was removed from the power position in her family. She would not have other opportunities to eat between scheduled meals and snacks no matter how upset she became and her own appropriate hunger pangs brought her to the table without negative behaviors or additional food strikes. Holly was receiving a great deal of attention for food refusal and the team encouraged the family to praise her enthusiastically for eating. Holly responded to attention for positive behaviors and negative behaviors decreased.

New foods were introduced and chains were written for each food Holly had eaten in the past as well as for crackers and juice. Milk intake was a major goal and the feeding specialist wrote a program to add orange sherbet and later Danimals Drinkable yogurt to juice to work toward acceptance of milk. A food/drink would be altered and then maintained at that level for three to four days to avoid shut down as Holly often reacted negatively to a change.

Transitions were extremely slow and gradual at first and Holly's parents required a great deal of encouragement to stay with the program, but as Holly began to make progress they felt they had turned a corner. Holly responded very well to additional treatment methods, especially with peer modeling and mealtime interaction at school. School personnel were educated regarding the treatment plan and followed the program as written. This patient demonstrated consistent success expanding food repertoire and additional food chaining programs were developed for introducing crunchy vegetables and fruits and treatment continued with modifying foods from all food groups.

Evaluation and Treatment of Pediatric Feeding Disorders: From NICU to Childhood

Holly's First Food Chain

Following is an example of a Food Chaining Calendar. Accepted foods and liquids are juice and crackers; first level of treatment.

Offer accepted juice with 5 small drops of pureed fruit mixed in (this is in attempt to change the texture of thin juice to a slightly thicker consistency)	No additional changes to juice today, hold this level, add two oyster crackers to saltines at snack. Repeat tomorrow.	Add 1-tsp. total of pureed fruit to juice today, mix well. Continue to add additional drops over the next three days. Then hold level.	Continue to add a variety of different crackers at snack time. Do not put the new crackers on her plate; just offer in a small bowel next to her plate to avoid refusals. Model eating new crackers.	Continue to offer new and preferred crackers by her plate. Add tiny dot of a slight film of butter to back on one of the saltine crackers.	Repeat plan today.	Offer new flavor of juice today. Continue with pureed fruit at same amount. Place one or two of the new crackers in the bowl on her plate. Add dot of peanut butter to back of one of the saltines.
Continue to alter juice with fruit smoothie (ice based) and offer crackers with butter and peanut butter in slightly larger amounts with a few plain crackers	Repeat plan today, but start offering a new food in the bowl beside her plate at each snack. Stay in the crunchy salty family, such as, Bugles, Tostitos, pretzel sticks (can dip in peanut butter) or potato chips.	Start adding 1/2 tsp. Danimals Drinkable yogurt to juice smoothie mix. This will begin our chain toward milk. If any resistance is observed, start with a **drop** and add a drop per day.	Continue to add Danimals yogurt to juice and increase amount daily through the weekend. Then stay at that level for three days.	Juice chain continues At PM snack offer one saltine cracker and a mix of new crunchy foods	Juice chain continues Repeat PM snack of one saltine and mix of new crunchy foods	Juice chain continues PM snack offer new crunchy foods only
Do not alter juice for next three days Offer mix of new crunchy foods at AM and PM snack	No changes	No changes	No changes	Offer juice with 1 T. or more if tolerated, Danimals Drinkable yogurt. Don't push it. Offer string cheese with crunchy foods at PM snack.	Offer chip dip in bowl beside plate. Model dipping crunchy snacks. Continue to offer string cheese, offer saltine today but increase butter or peanut butter amount.	Repeat plan next three days.
Hold	Hold	Hold	Offer baby carrots, crunchy snacks and string cheese with chip dip. 1/2 juice and 1/2 Danimals yogurt and hold through the weekend. Offer yogurt or ice-cream based fruit smoothie. No pressure.			New tastes to offer on plate: cheese quesadillas, cheese pizza, cheese and crackers and all other foods previously introduced. Continue peer/sibling modeling. Try strawberry milkshake before bed with curly straw.

104

Evaluation and Treatment of Feeding Aversion

Holly's Food Chain: Food Alteration Suggestions

Current/Past Foods	*Ways to alter current food into a new food*
Pancakes	Try a small amount (drops) of different flavor syrup over the regular syrup Put a small film of margarine under the syrup Buy a different brand or make homemade and freeze Make homemade in different shapes Add light powdered sugar Try French toast, French toast sticks, waffles mixed in with bites of pancakes Put a light smear of peanut butter on part of the pancake
Crackers	Buy a different brand, consider Goldfish, Oyster crackers, Club crackers, etc. Add a little seasoned salt, spray butter or garlic salt to 4-5 crackers, mix in with the rest
Pringles	Mix in a sour cream and onion Pringle or hide a small dot of chip dip on back side of one chip
Bread	Different brands, try homemade, rolls, breadsticks, bagels, pita bread, tortillas Toasted bread Garlic bread Add peanut butter/honey as tolerated
Dum Dum Sucker	Wet sucker and dust with small amount of flavored sugar (Lick 'em aide, pixie stix) in small area of sucker
Burger King French Fries	Sneak in one or two Ore Ida Fast Food fries Try other restaurants that have thin crispy style fries, such as, McDonald's, Sonic, Hardees or Steak and Shake Try Curly Fries Ketchup, mayo, ranch dressing offered for dipping. No pressure or just model it for her.
Juice	Blenderize in a small amount of orange sherbet and put in sippy cup (start modeling use of blender as we will transition to fruit smoothies when tolerated)
Milk (rarely accepted)	Add small amount of vanilla ice cream or flavored syrups (may just be a few drops at first) Add small amount of vanilla pudding
Popcorn	Spray a few kernels with Pam, add small amount of seasoned salt or Tabasco as she responds to strong flavor

Tips for Successful Food Chaining

- Determine which texture, consistency and flavor of food/liquid (if any) the child will accept. It is very important to transition to new foods and expand the food repertoire carefully, slowly and with a great deal of thought.
- With very sensitive children changes should be very gradual, with mild variations in taste, texture, consistency and temperature of foods.
- Do not push amounts, you want the child to try a new taste and feel comfortable. It may take several weeks to months to complete a chain.
- Offer foods the child feels comfortable with as well as a few bites of a new or transitional food. Many older children feel more comfortable if they can mask the flavor of a new food by alternating bites with comfort foods or with carbonated drinks. Put a bite of a new food with accepted foods early in the meal with young children, while they are hungry.
- With older children, encourage them to eat the new foods early in the meal and do not save it for the end. This can lead to an increase in refusals or negative experiences for the child.
- Tastes can be put on special spoons, curly straws, dippers or chopsticks, etc. Be creative and make it fun.
- Some children have the accepted food on their plate and may try 3-5 bites of the new or transitional food between bites of their favored item.
- Some children have difficulty moving from pureed foods to solids. To assist a child through this transition, try to remain in the same flavor family.

SAMPLE FOOD CHAIN

Transition Chain for Applesauce (Puree) to Solid

This chain was completed over a two-month time period. Very small changes occurred at first and the parents were cautioned to proceed very slowly. Restrictive feeding disorders take a long time to develop and a long time to extinguish. Gradually work down the list of foods to complete the food chain.

- Applesauce (currently an accepted food by the child) to
- Cinnamon Applesauce and regular applesauce mixed (1st change) to
- Cinnamon Applesauce (when accepted move to the next level) to
- Chunky Applesauce (alternate with smooth bites if needed, when accepted move to the next level) to
- Mashed cooked apples, with puree applesauce if needed, to
- Apple crisp or apple pie alternating with bites of puree or with ice cream to
- Apple crisp with tiny, thin pieces of raw apple added (when accepted move on) to
- Raw apple cut into small, narrow strips and dipped in applesauce to
- Thin, raw apple slices to
- Larger apple slices.

Evaluation and Treatment of Feeding Aversion

Transition Chain for Accepted Liquid Juice; Goal Liquid Milk

- Juice (currently accepted by the child) to
- All flavors of juice (first flavor change) to
- Juice smoothie-ice based (for first texture/temperature change) to
- Fruit smoothie-yogurt or ice cream based (for first milk-like flavor change) to
- Strawberry flavored milkshakes or for example, a Steak and Shake Fruit Freeze to
- Smooth fruit flavored yogurt (add real fruits as needed) to
- Ice Cream Sundae with fruit (for fading fruit taste out give occasional bites of ice cream only) to
- Vanilla milkshake to
- 1/2 shake and 1/2 milk to
- Regular milk.

What If the Child Refuses a Food in the Chain?

The therapist must think very carefully about foods recommended to try during the program. If a child refuses a new food, take a few steps backward until you find a way to present that flavor family or alter the consistency so the child is successful. Do not present endless choices or the child will keep manipulating the feedings. You may have to stay on one level of the food chain for a while before moving on. Make sure the transition is as smooth as possible. Stay away from large, hard chunks of a solid food. Make the lumps as small as possible.

With some very severe children, preferred foods may need to be altered so gradually that it takes weeks to months to complete a food chain. Refer to the food chain calendar for an example of a very slow moving food chain.

Older children can help develop their food chains and together the child and the therapists select foods to attempt that are similar to preferred or "comfortable" foods. For example, some children who are successful with spaghetti will try pizza because of the similarity of the sauce or a child, who will eat fish, may attempt shrimp or scallops.

Case Example: Eliot
Food Chaining for an Older Child; Feeding Aversion

History

This eleven year-old male had an unremarkable medical history. He started refusing foods at age two and over time developed a severely restricted food repertoire. At age eleven, he would eat only the center slices of a loaf of bread with peanut butter, a few "junk" foods that were crunchy, and he would drink milk, juice and soda. Milk intake was often excessive with 20 to 25 ounces at one time.

Eliot had one vomiting episode after staying with his grandparents; he felt pressured to eat a food outside his food repertoire and was taken to the emergency room due to the severity of the vomiting spell. He had a strong fear of vomiting and reported several choking spells. Eliot was also very aversive to the aroma of meat and stated that he needed to leave the house when his mother was cooking.

Evaluation

A complete evaluation by the pediatric feeding team revealed no underlying physical disorder or problem with the swallow. Weekly outpatient therapy was initiated. The team felt that long-term treatment was the best option to make a lasting change in Eliot's feeding behaviors.

Treatment Plan

Eliot was treated for his feeding disorder from July 2001 to September 2002. The therapist met with Eliot's parents prior to his initial visit to discuss the nature of the program and overall goals. The therapist felt that Eliot was very motivated to change his feeding behaviors because he wanted to go to camp and he was feeling increasing anxiety in social situations where food was involved. He felt the greatest stress at sleepovers and birthday parties. He was also referred for biofeedback therapy at the Center for Mind Body and Medicine at St. John's Hospital to address stress and anxiety from the challenges of the therapy program. Eliot attended sessions with his mother. Weekly sessions were scheduled and Eliot also contacted the therapist via voice mail reports 3-5 times weekly. A contract was written and signed by all parties at the end of each session and specific foods were targeted via food chaining.

Food Chaining Program

Eliot's preferred foods were analyzed and foods that were similar in texture, consistency and taste were selected off of those he felt successful with. Eliot used foods that he felt secure eating to alternate with new food items during his meals. Tastes of new foods were completed early in the meal as Eliot had a tendency to leave the new food for last and this made meals more difficult and stressful. Eliot was asked to rate foods by taste/texture on a scale from 1 to 10. Foods that were rated 4 or above were introduced again in a week or two. The therapist explained to Eliot that his tastes were changing and that he needed multiple exposures to new foods to rate them accurately.

Oral Sensory Brushing Program

An oral-sensory brushing program was also developed by the therapist for Eliot to complete daily. Eliot used an Infa-dent brush to complete the program as written by the therapist.

Motivation and Reinforcement

The therapist also wrote letters to Eliot to emphasize his progress and to share with other family members. Therapy sessions were fun and Eliot was motivated to attend. He had firm goals in mind related to his desire to go to camp. It was felt that this was critical to his success. The therapist also discussed Eliot's progress with his parents by phone and emphasized making sure that he did not feel a loss of attention from his family. Meals were no longer to focus on Eliot and this was a change in family dynamics. He needed to receive attention for schoolwork, athletic activities and other interests instead of receiving attention for not eating. It was felt that he might start seeking attention by sabotaging his feeding program. Eliot did have a behavioral component to his eating disorder and was close to inpatient admission in November of 2001. Family meetings as well as meetings with the therapist convinced Eliot to push through a difficult period in treatment and to continue to advance his goals. Holiday meals were targeted in treatment and Eliot ate the same meal as the rest of his family on Thanksgiving and Christmas.

Outcome

Soon through food chaining, he was eating a variety of all food groups and had mastered eating pizza and food items at most restaurants frequented by his family and friends. He was eating fruit and vegetable items and had achieved a level of success at breakfast and lunch meals. Focus of treatment turned to meats, dinner meals and the foods on the camp list.

Eliot met all goals in May of 2002 and in less than one year of treatment was eating a better than normal diet for an adolescent. He successfully attended football and youth camp and exceeded all goals for treatment.

Eliot's Advanced Food Chains
Accepted Food: Salad with ranch dressing

Later in our treatment program, Eliot found that he liked ranch dressing so we used it frequently in treatment to enhance the flavor of foods or mask newer tastes that he wasn't as comfortable eating. We used ranch dressing with salad and added increasing amounts of shredded vegetables, cheese, croutons (a favorite), and later started adding tiny pieces of boiled shrimp, crabmeat and eventually tiny pieces of deli-style turkey breast. This was a major accomplishment, as Eliot could not tolerate mixed consistencies of food in the beginning phases of treatment. Gradually, we increased the amount of meat in the salad. Chef style salads were quickly accepted with seafood and also tolerated fairly well with turkey. This was also a very healthy food choice and one that was easily accessible in any restaurant. Ham was rejected immediately and not felt to be a priority, so we negotiated to move to other meats. Chicken was introduced and again tolerated reasonably well. Eliot was advised to keep rotating the meats in his salads and that his tastes would continue to adapt and change. Taco salad was attempted but rated rather low on the numeric rating scale. He did agree to try it again, but beef was still rated low in taste and texture. We did not feel eating beef was necessary if Eliot was eating seafood and poultry. Salads were offered with hot rolls (a strong favorite and rolls were used as a transitional food that was comfortable and preferred). Breads were also chained to garlic bread, garlic biscuits, toasted bagels and cheese bread.

Later in the program, Eliot tried ranch dressing to mask the flavor of meats and found that adding them to his salad first was a great way to build his tolerance to other meats. As he adapted to the texture and taste of meat, we dipped pieces of seafood or chicken in small amounts of ranch dressing. Dressing was gradually faded from the meats so Eliot could adapt to the true flavor of the food item.

Eliot then began alternating bites of salad/bread/meat and gradually was able to eat larger portions of meat without the dipping technique. Seafood was selected first in the chain because it was rated highest and later became a favorite food. Seafood chaining continued and is described in the section below.

Meat Chain
Accepted Food: Fish (seasoned)

The first meat Eliot tolerated well was fried, seasoned fish in very thin slices. Additional seafood meat options that we explored included other types of fish, fried/broiled scallops, fried/broiled shrimp, crab-legs, and shrimp cocktail. This chain was developed later in the treatment program as Eliot initially had a strong aversion to meat. He did not like to chew meat and felt unsafe. He rejected all beef products, did not like chicken, but had a degree of success with fish at Red Lobster. He gave it a high number rating (6), so we tried to expand seafood choices in his diet. He assisted the therapist in developing a chain of food choices. We tried to remain as close to the accepted food as possible. He had great success with all of the foods in the chain, except for lobster. His mother wasn't too upset about that one! After developing a tolerance and preference for crunchy fish, he was able to transition to chicken strips as well. Chicken strips at Sonic were rated a nine on the one-ten scale and Eliot enjoyed going out to eat with his brothers and his friends at this restaurant.

For Parents: What is Food Chaining?

Food chaining, or taking liquids or foods your child currently accepts and linking those to similar liquids and foods, takes a great deal of thought. Some children have great anxiety with new foods or have a difficult time physically chewing the food and other children cannot tolerate the textures and tastes of new foods. This method eases children into new foods, without pressure and may help them through this transitional stage. Some children can only tolerate the slightest change at first and may respond best if new foods are offered one or two at a time and at snack times first. Your therapist and dietitian will customize food chains and methods of implementation for your child. The following are examples of a food chaining programs that may work for your child. These examples may start you thinking about what some of your goal foods are in effort to encourage your child to enjoy new food items.

REMEMBER

- A few bites of one new food are introduced at a time or as tolerated.
- Always give your child their primary or accepted food and put a few pieces of the new, targeted food in the chain on their plate or high chair tray.
- Do not force or push, model eating the new food and wait and see if the child attempts it from watching you.
- Do not tell your child to eat the new food, just offer it and see what happens. You may have to offer several times before the child will accept the new food. Some children will pick up a new food but not taste it. They are learning about the food by touching or smelling it and this should be considered an

110

initial success. Don't force the issue. Give it time and be patient. Steps may be small at first.

- New foods may be offered at snack times first if you feel your child will not tolerate changes easily. All foods in the chain have similarities in texture, consistency and/or flavor and each builds off the one before it. Do not break the chain or jump ahead.
- *This does not mean you cannot offer your child tastes or small portions of new foods.* The chains help guide you through flavor and texture families. New or surprise foods are encouraged once or twice a week. Your child may accept the new food especially in a new environment like a restaurant or friend's house. Food chains are not meant to limit you; they are a way to stop restricted mealtime behaviors.
- Have older kids rate foods on a scale from one to ten. Ten being the best. Offer foods again even if they are rejected. As your child's tastes adapt to new flavors, compare ratings. Often foods rated as a 4 or 5 one week, will be a 6 or 7 the next time they are tasted.
- Foods are listed in order of introduction in the chain. Your therapist will select specific foods for your child to master and will direct you how to offer foods successfully.

SAMPLE FOOD CHAINS

The child these four food chains were developed for accepted the following foods at the beginning of his treatment program: animal crackers, spaghettios, applesauce and juice.

At the beginning of the treatment program he had three foods and one liquid that he accepted. At the end of the food-chaining program he had close to thirty foods and seven liquids in his repertoire. The following chains were developed to expand his food repertoire and increase acceptance of foods of different flavors and textures.

ACCEPTED FOOD: ANIMAL CRACKERS
GOAL: EXPAND FOOD REPERTOIRE

This food chain took the accepted food and started adding foods that were also slightly sweet and crunchy, note that the it also introduces flavors of foods coming later in the chain. Peanut butter cookies introduced peanut butter crackers, Ritz and Club crackers maintained a slightly sweet taste but began the transition to salty flavor. Toast was introduced before bread because the child was most comfortable with crunchy foods. Additional food chains would then be added as each new flavor and texture was accepted. Cheese quesadillas could later be modified to add tiny pieces of chicken or grilled cheese could be introduced.

Food Chain Progression

- Animal Crackers (currently accepted) to
- Graham crackers
- Teddy Grahams
- Shortbread cookies
- Peanut butter cookies
- Club crackers to

- Cheese and crackers to
- Ritz crackers to oyster crackers to
- Saltine crackers to
- Cheese and crackers to
- Cheese quesadillas to
- Saltines with cheese or peanut butter to
- Toast with peanut butter or toasted cheese to
- Peanut butter and jelly sandwich

ACCEPTED FOOD: SPAGHETTIOS
Goal: Expand Food Repertoire

This food chain followed the child's preference for tomato-based sauce and built on pastas to advance the child to other Italian type foods. Chains may take some time to complete, but a child is much more likely to try a new food that is slightly familiar to him. Pizza can also be chained from breads/crackers.

Food Chain Progression

- Spaghettios (accepted by the child) to
- Variations of Spaghettios in different shapes to
- Chef Boyardee Ravioli to
- Spaghettios and/or Ravioli with small amount of regular spaghetti sauce mixed in to
- Spaghettios and/or Ravioli with macaroni noodles mixed in to
- Regular spaghetti to
- Lasagna or other pasta dishes/pizza.

ACCEPTED FOOD: APPLESAUCE
GOAL FOOD: APPLES (ADVANCING TEXTURE TO SOLIDS)

This chain is an example of staying with apple flavor and advancing texture of the food. Repeat with other flavors, such as, banana, peach, etc.

Food Chain Progression

- Applesauce (accepted food) to
- Other flavors of applesauce, such as Fruitsations Pear or Mango Applesauce
- Chunky applesauce (may have to fork mash chunks at first or cut into tiny slivers) to
- Chunky cinnamon or flavored applesauce to
- Soft apple slices of apple pie, fork mashed (may need to mix applesauce in with some children) to
- Larger pieces of baked apple or slices from apple pie (you may also try with ice cream to build on milk chain below) to
- Very thin slice of raw apple dipped in applesauce to
- Raw apple slice.

ACCEPTED LIQUID: JUICE
GOAL: LIQUID: MILK

A child may have developed a strong preference for juice or soda and may reject milk. Transitioning to milk is important; juice should be limited to 4 ounces a day. For some children it may take many months to work through this chain.

Liquid Chain Progression

- Juice to
- Different flavors/brands of juice to
- Juice with 1 teaspoon of orange sherbet or pureed fruit added to increase the consistency of the liquid to
- Juice with increased amount of pureed fruit or sherbet mixed in to
- Ice-based fruit smoothie to
- Ice based fruit smoothie with 1tablespoon Danimals drinkable yogurt to
- Fruit juice with increasing amounts of Danimals drinkable yogurt to
- Yogurt or ice cream based fruit smoothie to
- Strawberry milkshake to
- Strawberry milkshake/strawberry flavored milk (gradually thin out and increase milk) to
- Strawberry milk (gradually fade strawberry flavoring) to
- Regular milk and 2 tablespoons vanilla pudding added to
- Regular milk.

ADDITIONAL SUGGESTIONS

- No food should be pushed on the child. New foods should be offered in very small portions on the child's plate along with the foods that your child feels safe and comfortable eating.
- Do not tell young children to eat the new food, model eating it or let siblings/friends eat new foods during a snack with your child.
- Some children move very quickly through the initial food chains and others take a great deal of time to work through the first level of treatment. Be patient and stay on track.
- You can also offer novel foods to your child. Sometimes kids will surprise you and eat a new food the first time it is offered. Food chaining is not meant to limit what you can offer; it only serves as a method to expand foods following your child's known preferences. That is why we add "surprise foods" to the weekly program.
- Do not get into a habit of short order cooking with your children. The program will quickly move to the goal of incorporating foods from the family menu into your child's program. Our goal is that the entire family eats the same meal.
- Older children can be asked to try a new food and assured that it is very much like the foods they like. Older children can rate new foods on a scale from 1 to 10 according to taste and texture. Tastes will change, so offer targeted foods again and compare number ratings. They may change significantly. Pick foods that are rated 4 and up to offer again before foods that are in the 1 to 3 range.

Food Chain Calendar

Bread Products	Vegetables	Fruits	Meats	Dairy
Crackers	Green Beans	Apple	Hamburger	Milk
Bread	Peas	Banana	Roast beef (tender)	Ice Cream
Rolls	Corn	Orange	Sausage	Yogurt
Breadstick	Lettuce	Grapefruit	Hot dog (cut in	Cheese
Pita Bread	Broccoli	Cantaloupe	quarter strips)	Ice Milk
Flour Tortillas	Cauliflower	Watermelon	Pork	Cottage Cheese
Taco Shells	Tomato	Peaches	Turkey	
Pizza Crust	Sweet Potato	Kiwi	Chicken	
Flatbread	Baked Potato	Strawberry	Ham	
Biscuits	Squash	Cherries	Fish (check for	
Bun	Carrots	Tangerine	allergy)	
	Asparagus	Blueberries	Scallops	
	Black Eyed Peas	Blackberries	Shrimp	
		Nectarine	Crab	
		Pineapple	Veal	
		Grapes	Fowl	
		Raisins		
Condiments and Sauce	Convenience Foods	Other:	Other:	Other:
Mustard	Chicken Pot Pie			
Ketchup	TV Dinners			
A-1	(Salisbury steak,			
BBQ sauce	meatloaf, turkey)			
Worcestershire	Blenderize if			
Sauce	needed			
Soy Sauce	Spaghettios			
Salsa	Ravioli			
Taco Sauce	Beef Stew			
Sour Cream	(Blenderize if			
Butter	needed)			
Mayonnaise	Note: These are			
Salad Dressing	usually less			
Gravy	expensive and			
Cream soups	have stronger			
Cheese sauce	flavor than			
	Gerber Toddler			
	Meals			

Food Ideas for Families

Recommended consistency of food:

_____

_____

_____

_____

_____

Special Instructions:

_____

_____

_____

_____

_____

CHAPTER NINE
▲
Special Topics

Special topics are designed to be a quick reference guide for the busy therapist. We have had many experiences where we had five minutes to run to a book and look something up. We wrote this section to give a quick, yet detailed overview of diagnosis, treatment and referral considerations to the therapist on the go.

Chat Time

Remember when working with children who have special needs, focus on the child. Research the diagnosis and make sure you are looking thoroughly at the child, but don't lose focus on the feedings. Assess feeding disorders as you would in any child. See where there are problems and start forming a treatment plan to improve the child's skills. We tell our students to "become the child," see what the child is doing and mimic it, this will teach you a great deal about the child's oral movement patterns as well as the feeding disorder. Many of the traditional oral motor therapy techniques work with children who fall into the special topics category, however, we encourage you to be creative and let the children have fun during treatment. Oral sensory motor programs should also be explored to teach the child about the mouth.

Cleft Lip and Palate

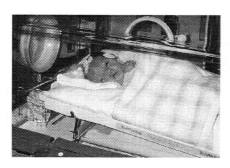

POSITIONING SUPPORT

An upright, sidelying positioning for the infant will help to decrease nasopharyngeal reflux and assist in bolus control as the milk collects in the buccal area prior to entering the pharynx. Provide jaw and cheek support.

EVALUATION

Assess oral reflexes and the degree of the cleft and use cervical auscultation to check the swallow. Consider an ENT referral if not completed. The ENT should check for soft palate function, vocal cord closure and rule out laryngeal cleft.

REDUCING INTAKE DEMANDS

If weight gain is a concern, concentrated formula feedings will reduce intake demands and provide adequate caloric intake.

FEEDING METHODS

Breastfeeding can be a good option for cleft lip/palate babies as the breast-tissue helps fill the cleft and increase negative pressure in the oral cavity. A supplemental nursing system (SNS) and nipple shield should improve breastfeeding success.

The Pigeon Nipple/bottle is the best product we have found for cleft lip/palate babies, however, it may be too large for premature infants. Depending on the type and extent of the cleft, The Dr. Brown Bottle with the Y-cut nipple with a smaller amount of cereal is another option for cleft palate babies.

The cleft palate nurser bottle can be used with the Ross Orthodontic nipple, which is a high flow nipple; however, this is a disposable product and must be ordered by the case for home use. (Use high flow because of the infant's decreased intra-oral pressure, but assess swallow carefully). Ross nipple also contains latex. Repair is usually at 10 pounds or around 3 months of age for lip and 12-18 months for palate. Cleft palate nurser can also be used with more standard type nipples, but look carefully at how the milk leaves the nipple when pressure is applied to the cleft palate squeeze bottle. You do not want the milk to shoot out with force into the pharynx. Place the nipple under the most intact section of palate.

SPOON FEEDING

Older infants (6 months) may benefit from using the pacifier as the first spoon or alternating spoon and pacifier to help clear the oral cavity. In addition, older children benefit from mouthing programs and oral sensory motor therapy for speech production as well as for feeding.

Tracheomalacia and Laryngomalacia

TRACHEOMALACIA: DEFINITION AND ETIOLOGY

- Tracheomalacia is a disorder of the trachea that causes it to be abnormally collapsible due to the loss of structural integrity.
- Tracheal rings are soft and cannot prevent the airway from collapsing especially during exhalation. The entire cartilaginous structure of the upper airway may be involved or it may be a localized area of decreased rigidity.
- It may be due to abnormal development of the foregut and vasculature in embryonic life or may be seen with vascular anomalies such as vascular ring, esophageal atresia and TE fistula. Can also result from internal compression from an endotracheal tube or tracheotomy tube.
- Diffuse malacia may be congenital and associated with no other anomalies. As the child grows, structural integrity is gradually restored.

Special Topics

CHARACTERISTICS AND FEEDING CHALLENGES

Tracheomalacia is characterized by noisy respirations and expiratory stridor. Generally symptoms are present at birth. Hoarseness, aphonia and inspiratory retractions may be present and serious enough to cause chest wall deformity. Infant/child will have problems with coordination of the suck/swallow/breathe sequence. Poor weight gain may also be a complication.

Laryngomalacia: Definition and Etiology

Laryngomalacia is collapse of the supraglottic laryngeal structures. Symptoms are present during inspiration as the epiglottis or aryepiglottic folds may be pulled into the airway during inspiration. Diagnosis is based on bronchoscopy findings.

TREATMENT OPTIONS

- Treatment includes position change during feeding and feeding the infant slowly. Rarely do children need a tracheotomy.
- Long term prognosis is good.
- Refer or consult with occupational or physical therapy for assistance with positioning.
- Carefully select a nipple for this patient and make sure flow rate is appropriate for the entire feeding.
- Watch for signs of fatigue with feeding.
- Modified barium swallow study is recommended. Use cervical auscultation to monitor the patient's swallow during feeding sessions.

Down Syndrome

INCIDENCE AND CHARACTERISTICS

Approximately one out of every 800 to 1100 births results in Trisomy 21 or Down Syndrome, and about 40% to 50% are born with some type of cardiac abnormality. A large percentage develop Mitral Valve Prolapse by adulthood. Most have a compromised immune system with a corresponding decrease in the number of T cells is a characteristic of most individuals with Down Syndrome.

COMPLICATIONS

- Rate of infection is higher and patients have an extremely high incidence of peridontal disease. (Leonard, Leonard, Petterson, Bower)
- Chronic upper respiratory infections are associated as many of the children are mouth breathers and have xerostomia (dry mouth) with fissuring of the tongue and lips, aphthous ulcers, oral candida infections and acute necrotizing ulcerative gingivitis. Mouth breathing may also decrease saliva in the oral cavity and increase risk of dental caries.
- There is an increased risk of sleep apnea.

118

- True macroglossia is rare, rather a relative macroglossia is present where the tongue is of normal size but the oral cavity is reduced due to underdevelopment of the midface.

STRUCTURAL VARIATIONS

- Eruption of teeth may be delayed and occur in an unusual order, some teeth may be missing.
- Reduced muscle tone affects the musculature of the head and oral cavity as well as the large skeletal muscles. Reduced tone in the cheeks and lips contribute to an imbalance of the forces on the teeth with the force of the tongue being a greater influence. This contributes to the open bite often seen in these children.

ORAL PERIPHERAL EXAMINATION

- Less efficient chewing and natural cleansing of the teeth (more material remains on the surfaces of the teeth) may also contribute to increased peridontal disease.
- Abnormalities in orofacial structures (hypoplasia of the midfacial region with smaller bones of the midface and maxilla) can cause occlusion abnormalities.
- Tend to have a high and vaulted palate.

TREATMENT OPTIONS

- Breastfeeding is possible and very good for the baby. Special alerting and positioning techniques, oral exercises prior to feeding, upright positioning, frequent burp breaks may help the baby.
- For bottle-feeding, use higher-flow nipples. (Note: Assess swallow function!) This may decrease fatigue, and/or nipples that help with lip seal may improve feeding and decrease air intake. You also want a nipple that provides input to midline tongue to encourage tongue grooving and improve bolus control. The babies tend to rapidly imprint on the first nipple introduced.
- Develop an oral motor program to build muscle tone and improve tongue positioning at rest.
- Speech therapy should continue to follow the infant consistently for oral motor therapy, monitoring of feeding skills and language stimulation.
- Oral sensory motor treatment is strongly recommended.

Cardiac Conditions

Please note: Many cardiac patients can feed well, but lack endurance to take a sufficient amount of formula/food in a timely manner. Cardiac patients require special nutritional care from a pediatric dietitian. Concentrated feedings may be needed as these patients burn calories at a higher rate. Concentrated feedings decrease the amount of formula the baby needs to nipple per feeding and may improve over-all endurance.

High flow nipples often work well with cardiac patients, but *thoroughly* assess the swallow prior to making this recommendation to the family. Assess

Special Topics

the entire feeding due to fatigue issues, which may lead to an increased risk of aspiration. Treat for endurance problems and try to make intake as effortless as possible.

A modified barium swallow study or FEES may be indicated. Occupational therapy is also recommended to assist in treatment and treat children post-operatively who will need special attention in regard scar care, development of motor skills and assessment for sensory dysfunction.

The following are descriptions of some of the cardiac conditions seen in preemies and newborns.

PATENT DUCTUS ARTERIOSUS

The ductus arteriosus, an extra blood vessel in the heart before birth, fails to close after birth. Blood from the aorta continues to flow through it into the pulmonary artery, so excess blood passes through the lung vessels. Can cause shortness of breath during the exertion of feeding. Often closes on it's own or is closed surgically later in life.

COARCTATION OF THE AORTA

Coarctation of the aorta is a localized narrowing of the aorta that reduces the supply of blood to the lower part of the body. Symptoms include headaches, weakness on exertion, weak or absent pulses in the groin, and coldness in the legs. High blood pressure above the narrowed area and low blood pressure below it occurs and if the aorta is extremely constricted, severe heart failure occurs. May have congestive heart failure with hepatomegaly. Surgery is necessary in all cases later in life.

TETRALOGY OF FALLOT

Four abnormalities occur together including hole in the upper ventricular septum, a displacement of the aorta to the right so that blood from both ventricles enters it, pulmonary stenosis, and a thickening of the right ventricle wall. Cyanosis, clubbing of the fingers and toes, and underdevelopment occur. After exercise the child is short of breath and squats to relieve discomfort. Surgery should be carried out before the child is five years old.

TRANSPOSITION OF THE GREAT VESSELS

The aorta and the pulmonary arteries are transposed, so that oxygenated blood from the lungs passes through the pulmonary artery and back to the lungs, instead of through the aorta and to the tissues. Unless there is a hole in the septum or some other passageway that allows some of the oxygenated blood to pass into the right side of the heart and the aorta, the baby will not survive. See cyanosis, clubbing and underdevelopment. In all cases emergency surgery creates a larger hole in the septum before the baby is three months old. A second operation is completed before the child is five years old.

CONGENITAL AORTIC STENOSIS

A narrowing near the beginning of the aorta, and sometimes the aortic valve as well, that restricts the flow of blood to the body. Usually no effects until later, in some rare cases the child has shortness of breath, chest pain and blackouts. Surgery is done later in life to relieve or remove the constriction.

CONGENITAL PULMONIC STENOSIS

Congenital pulmonic stenosis is a narrowing of the pulmonary valve or more rarely, the upper right ventricle, that reduces blood flow to the lungs. Shortness of breath on exertion, cyanosis, may be severe heart failure. Surgery needed in moderate or severe cases.

VENTRICULAR SEPTAL DEFECT

This is the most common of all congenital heart diseases. Characterized by a hole in the ventricular septum or wall, usually the upper part. Blood flows abnormally from the left ventricle to the right, sometimes in large quantities, so that excess blood passes through the lung vessels, which are served in this chamber. If VSD is severe, the baby may tire easily and have shortness of breath on exertion. Occasionally there is severe heart failure or pulmonary hypertension. A larger hole requires surgery but a smaller one usually does not require treatment.

ATRIAL SEPTAL DEFECT

This is a hole in the atrial septum or wall. Blood passes from the left atrium into the right, sometimes in large amounts so that excess blood circulates through the lungs. Child may have increased risk of failure to thrive and recurrent respiratory infections. Most babies have no symptoms, but some tire and have shortness of breath and pulmonary hypertension can develop. Surgically treated unless the hole is very small and there is minimal risk of pulmonary hypertension developing later in life.

Extracorpreal Membrane Oxygenation (ECMO)

An ECMO machine is very similar to a heart-lung bypass machine. A child is placed on ECMO and their blood receives oxygenation from an artificial lung in the ECMO pump. This will provide the child with oxygen needed to live until their lungs are able to function well enough to sustain life. The blood containing very little oxygen is drained via gravity from the patient from a catheter placed in a large vein in the neck. The pump will push the blood through the ECMO system. Blood will be cleansed of carbon dioxide and pick up oxygen. Once the blood is oxygenated it is warmed and returned to the child through the arterial catheter.

Hypoxic-Ischemic Encephalophathy (HIE)

DEFINITION, ETIOLOGY, AND CHARACTERISTICS

Term infant with history of perinatal asphyxia that exhibits clinical signs of acute brain injury. HIE is also seen with multisystem disease. It may occur due to abruptio placentae or from umbilical cord compression, or, it may also occur in older children due to asphyxia or multisystem disease. With *mild encephalopathy* the infant may present with maximum presentation of symptoms in the first 24 hours post-partum. Improvement may be seen by one-week of age. Characteristics include brief lethargy, jitteriness, hyper-alert state, irritability, hyper-responsiveness to stimulation, tachycardia, dilatation of pupils, transient hypoglycemia, and decreased secretions.

- *Moderate encephalopathy* has a critical period of 48 to 72 hours post-partum. There is either improvement or the infant deteriorates. Improvement is indicated by no further seizure activity, transient jitteriness and an improving level of consciousness. Deterioration is indicated by seizures, cerebral edema, lethargy and abnormal EEG results. Characteristics include lethargy, hypotonia, decreased spontaneous movement, jitteriness and discrepant muscle strength between the shoulder and pelvic regions.

- *Severe encephalopathy* presents with a level of consciousness that deteriorates from obtunded to stupor to comatose. Mechanical ventilation is required to sustain life. Characteristic features include: apnea, seizures appearing within the first 12 post-natal hours, tonic and multifocal seizures within the first day of life, severe hypotonia, absent reflexes, Doll's eye movements, present and reactive pupils. If the infant deteriorates, over 24 to 72 hours the pupils become unreactive, seizure activity increases, cerebral edema occurs, the EEG shows burst-suppression pattern and death may ensue. Long-term sequelae are based on site and extent of cerebral injury. (Beachy and Deacon, 1993)

COMPLICATIONS

The infant may experience an increased risk of gastroesophageal reflux, increased risk of seizures, dysphagia, tone issues, or severe developmental delay.

TREATMENT

- Infant/child may present with hypersensitivity in the peri-oral region and hyposensitivity in the intra-oral/pharyngeal region. Child will benefit from an oral sensory motor program to attempt to normalize sensation in the oral facial region.
- Modified barium swallow is indicated prior to oral intake.
- Infants/children who aspirate may need a direct thermal stimulation program to improve swallow function and improve intra-oral/pharyngeal awareness.
- The infant/child may respond best to strong flavors or chilled foods and liquids.
- Paired oral motor feeding and oral sensory motor treatment programs are recommended.
- Co-treatment with occupational therapy should be completed when possible.

Shaken Baby Syndrome and Brain Injury

"Current data suggests that, even in adults, sensory stimulation may facilitate brain remodeling to facilitate swallowing after brain injury. Also, continuing oral stimulation will prevent the development of aversion to oral touch, allowing good dental care."
--Hamdy S, et al: Organization and reorganization of human swallowing motor cortex: Implications for recovery after stroke. Clin Sci 99:151-157, 2000.

DEFINITION OF SHAKEN BABY SYNDROME

Due to their irritability and higher degree of care needs, preemies are at high risk for being victims of shaken baby syndrome. Shaken Baby Syndrome is defined as rigorous shaking of an infant or small child usually for 5-20 seconds with a rotational or angular force forward and backward, bouncing the brain within the skull, often ending in a forceful blunt trauma to the head by impact on a surface.

DEFINITION OF TRAUMATIC BRAIN INJURY

TBI may be open head injury, closed head injury, blunt trauma or hypoxic injury.

TEAM INTERVENTION PROGRAM

The patient will require team intervention from pediatrics, nursing, rehab medicine, neurology, gastroenterology, PT/OT/ST, dietitian, child life, social work, respiratory therapy and other specialists as needed. Counseling and support should be provided as needed to the child, family or foster care providers as needed.

The school district should be notified upon admission to the hospital and team members from the hospital and the school should start forming the treatment program.

DEFICIT AREAS

- Injuries received from SBS are similar to that of a closed head injury/TBI which includes injury resulting in impairments to one or more areas such as: cognition, language, memory, attention, reasoning, abstract thinking, judgment, problem-solving, sensory, perceptual, motor abilities, psycho-social behavior, physical functions, information processing and speech.
- Range of injury can be mild to extreme.
- Retinal damage is also seen in infants with SBS.
- Risk of seizure activity following SBS is very high and can impact swallow function.

EVALUATION STRATEGIES

- Initial assessment of a patient suffering from SBS should include examination of oral motor functioning.

Special Topics

- Patient may not have the ability to suck or swallow appropriately. In these cases, the speech pathologist will work to help re-organize the patient's oral motor skills and determine when and if the patient is safe for oral feedings.
- Some techniques to help the patient increase awareness of their oral peripheral mechanism for mechanics such as sucking and swallowing include the following:

    1. Firm proprioceptive input to all four quadrants of the gum ridge may facilitate the patient's awareness and organization of their oral structures.
    2. Firm pressure to the hard palate may increase the patient's awareness of their structures and facilitate a sucking pattern.
    3. A chilled pacifier may increase the patient's awareness of objects within the oral cavity and facilitate sucking response.
    4. Stroking the faucial arches with an iced gloved finger or giving drops of chilled formula while the infant is sucking on the finger or chilled pacifier may increase pharyngeal awareness for a patient with a delayed swallow reflex.
    5. Tastes of lemon juice or other strong flavors on a pacifier or gloved finger may increase awareness and help prepare the patient for feeding.

- A speech and language evaluation also should be completed to determine the patient's current level of function and to design a treatment program with other members of the team.
- This evaluation can be compared to previous level of function (via parental report or past medical history) to determine degree of loss.
- Re-evaluation should be completed annually. TBI and SBS affect the patient's new learning skills.

TREATMENT

Please note: Once the patient is able to take small amounts of food orally, a modified barium swallow study is indicated. Usually a series of swallow studies is needed, especially in the acute stage. Additional assessments will be needed with changes in tone or with significant growth.

- Even if the infant or child appears to be feeding well, status can change suddenly.
- Continue to aggressively monitor intake and daily status. Talk to the physician and nursing staff about any oral medications ordered for the patient due to risk of aspiration.
- Long-term care and environmental support.
- It is critical that the patient receives intensive rehabilitative treatment for at least the first year post-injury, as this is the time the majority of gains can be achieved. Strategies to assist the patient with language skills and new learning strategies should be incorporated into the program.
- Family care needs include support systems for school transition and individual education programming, counseling, education regarding long term needs and ongoing treatment programs.

124

Seizure Disorder

ETIOLOGY AND OUTCOME

Seizures result from excessive simultaneous electrical discharge or depolarization of neurons. They may result from metabolic encephalopathies, IVH, trauma, HIE, infection, withdrawal from maternal drugs or they may be genetic in nature. Treatment and outcome is related to etiology. (Beachy and Deacon, 1993)

SEIZURE DISORDER AND FEEDING SKILLS

Subtle or marked differences in feeding behaviors may be observed after seizure activity. Re-assess skills after any change in status, especially after reports of feeding differences by caregivers. Oral-motor feeding and oral sensory-motor programs are recommended, as should a Modified Barium Swallow study or FEES be completed.

TYPES OF SEIZURES

- Subtle seizures are the most frequent neonatal seizures and are often unrecognized. Presentation varies: horizontal deviation of the eyes, pedaling movements, swimming movements, eye blinking or fluttering, non-nutritive sucking, smacking lips, drooling and apnea.
- Tonic seizures are characteristic in premature infants weighing less than 2500 grams. Often seen with severe IVH and the infant may present with generalized tonic extension of all extremities or flexion of upper limbs with extension of lower extremities and may mimic decorticate posturing.
- Multifocal seizures are characteristic in full-term infants with HIE, may see clonic movement patterns that migrate from one limb to another without a specific pattern.
- Focal clonic seizures are uncommon and present as localized jerking.
- Myoclonic seizures are very rare in the neonatal period and are characterized by multiple jerks of upper or lower limb flexion.

Cerebral Palsy

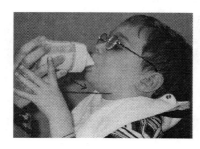 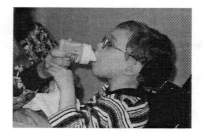

These photos were taken after Christopher was evaluated in wheelchair clinic. Both demonstrate his skills for drinking liquid from a cup. The left picture shows poor positioning with head hyperextension and tightness in his oral musculature and through the larynx. The speech pathologist worked with the seating and mobility team to make adjustments to his chair. Once the adjustments were made, his head was in a more neutral position and the tightness diminished.

Special Topics

Fully evaluate feeding and swallowing skills. Develop a feeding program with the family and set appropriate goals. Initially the child may be NPO, so focus therapy on improving secretion management, development of oral skills and direct swallow therapy if appropriate. If the child can orally feed, determine what foods and liquids are safe.

ASSESS CALORIC NEEDS AND MAXIMUM INTAKE POTENTIAL

A pediatric dietitian should assess intake via food logs and determine with the feeding therapist energy expenditure to complete a meal or snack. A co-evaluation with an occupational or physical therapy is strongly recommended to assist the feeding therapist with positioning and seating options. Optimal positioning will give you an idea of the amount of food a child can safely consume for one meal. Carefully assess the child's positioning of the neck and shoulder girdle. The feeding specialist should participate in wheelchair clinics when possible to assess positioning for secretion management as well as oral feedings.

EVALUATION AND TREATMENT STRATEGIES

- Assess for safest consistencies of liquid and food, complete a MBS or FEES to completely assess feeding skills and rule out silent aspiration.
- Many children with cerebral palsy respond best to strong flavors, consider adding seasoning, such as: A-1 sauce, garlic, taco seasoning, jerk seasoning, seasoned salt, ketchup, salsa, mustard, mayo to pureed meats; sherbet, pudding, carbonation, flavored sauces to liquids, butter, chicken broth, mushroom gravy to vegetables to increase sensory feedback and improve flavor. Experiment with a variety of seasoning choices; however, leave some foods bland as the child will habituate to flavoring if all foods are highly seasoned.
- Oral hygiene and oral motor exercise programs should be taught to caregivers as part of activities of daily living.
- Cotton candy and Pixie Stix powder are good choices for oral exercise programs due to strong flavor and no bolus to swallow.
- Oral sensory motor programs are very important when working with children with cerebral palsy. Age appropriate teether or mouthing type toys should be used when working with children with cerebral palsy.
- Use a mirror when completing oral sensory or oral-motor feeding programs, so the child can observe movements of the structures. Tell the child what you are doing and what you want him to do with his body. Give the child as much feedback as possible.

A Word About Thickened Liquids

Many children require thickened liquids, however, commercial thickening agents may increase constipation, are not consistent feeding to feeding due to inconsistencies in amount given from feeder to feeder and consistency changes as the thickening agent remains in the liquid. Taste is also a factor in that some children will reject thickened liquids and have insufficient liquid intake. Parents/caregivers may forget or not like dealing with Thick-It or Thick'em Up and periodically give thin liquids increasing risk of aspiration. Following are some alternatives to Thick It or Thick'em Up:

- Milk or Pediasure thickened with pudding packs or with ice cream and/or Carnation Instant Breakfast Powder (great calorie booster). Generally speaking, 4 ounces of milk/pediasure can be thickened with 2-8 ounces of pudding. Thicken according to the child's needs. This mixture can be easily stored in a thermos or container and can be used by the parent throughout the day. Shake well prior to use.

- Juice thickened with orange sherbet or pureed fruit (applesauce in apple juice). Recipe is 4 ounces of juice with 4 to 10 ounces of pureed fruit. Again the therapist must determine the consistency needed for safe swallowing.

- Orange Juice/Orange Sherbet/7up works well to clear the pharynx as it does not coat the throat and is great for oral alerting or to use to clear between bites of thicker foods. Mix ingredients to the proper consistency. This mixture should not be stored and must be prepared at the meal.

- Yogurt or fruit smoothies (add Danimals Drinkable Yogurt to liquids or combine Yoplait Custard Style Yogurt, fresh fruit, juice and CIB powder in blender).

REMEMBER

Measure amounts needed to thicken liquids per child's need and write "recipes" for family. These methods of thickening remain consistent throughout the meal, increase calories and provide improved flavor of liquids. They can also be prepared ahead of meal times and stored in containers (shake well) for easy use throughout the day.

The right consistency of liquid can reduce the risk of aspiration. These calorically dense drinks are also a great option for the child who needs a high calorie intake program.

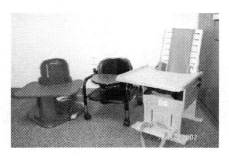

▲ *Corner, ladybug, and theradapt chirs* ▲

Corner, ladybug, and theradapt chairs are just a few examples of positioning devices that may be used during feedings. Collaboration between an occupational therapist and speech therapist will determine how positioning of the body affects the tone of the oral musculature and swallowing.

Special Topics

Esophageal Atresia and Tracheoesophageal Fistula

INCIDENCE, ETIOLOGY AND TYPES OF FISTULAS

- Incidence varies between 1 in 800 and 1 in 5000 live births; 30% to 40% of affected infants have associated anomalies (cardiac defects and imperforate anus are most common).
- Types include: esophageal atresia with tracheoesophageal fistula, isolated esophageal atresia, H-type tracheoesophageal fistula and esophageal atresia with upper pouch fistula.
- Clinical presentation is dependent on the type of tracheal/esophageal anomaly. The infant cannot manage secretions; the gastric tube cannot be passed, choking or cyanosis is observed with the initial feeding attempt.
- May have a history of polyhydramnois.

TREATMENT

- Surgical repair is needed. Postoperative complications include respiratory distress, pneumonia, sepsis, dismotility of the lower esophageal segment and unilateral diaphragmatic paralysis.
- Dilatation of the esophagus may be necessary if anastomotic stricture occurs.
- Infants may have stridor or "brassy" cough from tracheomalacia. Occasionally, this is severe enough to require a tracheotomy.
- Gastroesophageal reflux is common. The child may also have esophageal motility issues as a result of this disorder.

Autistic Spectrum Disorder

REMEMBER

For children with autistic spectrum disorder refer to the feeding aversion chapter and use food-chaining techniques to gradually expand the child's food repertoire. PECS or ABA style intervention strategies can be easily applied to feeding programs when working with these challenging patients.

Remember, the basics still apply here; stimulate appetite; help the child interpret the sensation of hunger and associate it with the act of eating through concrete language and a predictable chain of events; find the foods the child is comfortable eating and gradually adjust those foods in the same flavor and texture family to expand the food repertoire; and follow the child's cues to keep expanding the diet.

Consultation with an occupational therapist and pediatric dietitian are strongly recommended. Watch these children for constipation problems as this can significantly impact nutritional intake.

STRUCTURING THE FEEDING ENVIRONMENT

- Changes to their diet may be very distressing for the child and there is a risk of complete food refusal.

- Structure the mealtime routine so the child knows what to expect and feels as secure as possible. Consistent, concrete language is recommended.
- Picture schedules/choice boards may help some children at mealtime.

SENSORY PROCESSING DISORDERS AND RESTRICTED FOOD REPERTOIRE

Children with autistic spectrum disorder often have sensory processing problems and have a very restricted food repertoire.

- Food chaining is strongly recommended with very gradual, minor changes to foods.
- Move to new foods in the same flavor family.
- Some children with autism do well finger-feeding so they receive sensory input about the texture of a bite of food before placing it in the mouth.
- Some children with autism like to drink from a sip-cup for oral input and organization, if they are drinking juice they will significantly dampen their appetite.
- If the child needs to cup from a sensory standpoint, put water in the cup instead of juice. Or gradually dilute the juice to water. Consult an occupational therapist for sensory based alternatives to cup drinking.
- Some children with autism do not associate hunger pangs and eating, they may show distress or act out as a result. Scheduled meals and snacks are strongly recommended.

INTERNAL MOTIVATION

Appetite is key to improving intake. Make sure the child has opportunities for play and activity that will stimulate appetite (supervised water-play or swimming, if tolerated by the child, are good choices). Vitamin supplements are a good recommendation for children with autism.

GLUTEN CASEIN FREE DIETS

For most people, the breakdown of dietary protein into smaller and smaller proteins and finally into individual amino acids is a process that is smoothly completed as food travels through the digestive system. However, for an autistic individual, it has been proposed that a defect in the intestinal wall permits incompletely digested components of the original proteins to pass from the intestine into the bloodstream.

In the case of two of the diet's most common proteins, gluten (from wheat, barley, oats, and rye) and casein (from milk), some of the components that are released into the bloodstream have opioid (morphine-like) properties. Gliadorphin-7 and other similar polypeptides are formed in the breakdown of gluten. Bovine ß-casomorphin-7 and other similar polypeptides are formed in the breakdown of casein.

Most recently, deltorphin and dermorphin have been targeted for their potential activity as well. All of these polypeptides contain regions very similar in structure to morphine. The theory is these proteins are transported to the brain where they bind to receptors causing an effect that some research indicates is manifested in the symptoms of autism.

Special Topics

Some children show a marked difference in their behavior and language when gluten and casein free diets are implemented.

A pediatric dietitian should be consulted to assist families who wish to eliminate gluten and casein from their child's diet.

Cancer

Children with cancer can develop feeding aversion secondary to nausea and vomiting from chemotherapy.

- Relaxation therapy may help with nausea.
- Needs vary according to the type of cancer.
- A side effect of chemotherapy is sores inside the mouth. There are programs to help reduce symptoms and to assist with oral care; this is usually managed by the oncologist or RN.
- Infa-dents and Toothettes for oral care may be easier on delicate tissue.
- Hydration is very important, as the chemo destroys cancer cells; toxins are released into the system. If the child does not have adequate intake of fluids, the toxins accumulate causing more nausea in a cyclic pattern.
- Children should take liquids by straw when possible. This will increase the volume and reduce air intake. Generally encourage 1/2 cup of liquid per 30 minutes if possible.
- Calorically dense drinks (see recipes for thickened liquids in CP section) or supplements such as Pediasure, KinderCal, ScandiShakes or NuBasics juice may be beneficial if tolerated.
- Reward systems, motivators are important to encourage adequate fluid intake.
- If the child tolerates water, try liquids with a few calories such as diluted juice.
- Some children with cancer benefit from g-tube placement.
- Consult with a pediatric dietitian is recommended.
- Medical staff, child life specialists, tutors/school personnel and rehab therapists should meet to develop a comprehensive care plan for the child.

CHAPTER TEN

▲

Nutrition and Digestive Tract Disorders

Nutrition Problems and Digestive Disorders

Why does a feeding specialist need to know about disorders of the GI tract and digestive problems? A feeding specialist takes a detailed history prior to working with a patient and the patient's family has time to talk about their child's feeding patterns in great detail. The therapist may gather valuable information in these discussions with the family that will assist the team or physician to determine contributing factors to the feeding disorder.

The therapist should always ask about tube feeding schedules and practices, formula type and use, GI discomfort associated with feeding, constipation, reflux, vomiting and weight gain. Digestive tract disorders or discomfort after feeding can result in poor oral intake, poor weight gain and inadequate hydration. Many times these problems are at the core of a child's feeding problem.

The Digestive Tract

THE MOUTH

Food is in the mouth for approximately one minute and the teeth, tongue and saliva break down food as ptyalin enzymes convert starch into maltose and dextrose soluble sugars ready for digestion.

THE STOMACH

Food stays here two to four hours, churns and mixes the food and hydrochloric acid kills bacteria and protease enzymes break down protein

THE SMALL INTESTINE

Includes the duodenum, jejunum and ileum. The duodenum is very short and receives digestive enzymes from the pancreas and bile from the liver and gall bladder (storage). The digestive juices break down the food. The major part of digestion and absorption of nutrients takes place in the jejunum. Food stays here approximately 1 to 6 hours, the small intestine walls and pancreas secrete amylase, protease, and lipase enzymes into the lumen to digest starch, fats and protein. The gall bladder secretes bile to emulsify fats and break them down to hydrochloric acid from the stomach as the small intestine works in an alkaline

131

pH. Once secretions have reduced all the nutrients to molecule size, they are absorbed into the blood stream through the epithelial cells of the millions of villi. Villi are rich in blood vessels and give the walls of the small intestine a huge surface area, approximately that of a tennis court. This enables sufficient absorption of micronutrients necessary for life. Indigestible material, soluble and insoluble as well as waste by-products of the digestive process is evacuated into the last stage.

THE LARGE INTESTINE OR COLON

Products remain here two hours to days. The large intestine contains millions of live active bacteria, which aid in the breakdown to form waste products. Water is absorbed along with electrolytes and waste material passes out via the rectum.

Non-Oral Feeding

Tube feedings (nasogastric, orogastric, gastric) may be recommended to enhance weight gain or to increase the nutritional status of an infant who aspirates or does not have the endurance to meet nutritional needs via oral feedings. A feeding tube should not be considered an "either or" method of nutrition, unless the child is aspirating and unsafe for oral feedings. In these cases, direct swallowing therapy and thermal stimulation techniques should be implemented to try to regain swallowing function and nutritional intake should be through a feeding tube.

A feeding tube can be used in many ways to supplement oral feeding, for example, for some children, overnight drip feedings can be given and the child can eat orally during the day or the child may receive a smaller bolus after each meal.

If the child is ill, a feeding tube is very valuable and reduces pressure on the family until the child recovers and can resume partial oral intake. Families may need a support person or counseling to help them realize that for their child, alternative approaches to providing nutritional support may be better for the child's overall health and reduce the time providing nutrition to allow for other nurturing activities.

Hydration issues can be addressed with a feeding tube as many special needs children do not have sufficient fluid intake. If the child is adequately hydrated constipation problems may also be reduced. Medications can also be given through the g-tube helping the parent get a consistent dosage in the child each time.

A nasogastric tube can be used for short-term non-oral intake. If a child will not be able to meet nutritional needs orally for three to four months or more, a g-tube should be considered. Issues to consider with feeding tubes include:

THERAPY PROGRAMS

- Oral motor therapy is vital to help the child preserve their sucking and swallowing patterns and normal sensation.
- Therapy programs should provide as many positive oral experiences as possible.

Nutrition and Digestive Disorders

- Therapy programs should focus on reducing negative oral experiences, assessing and improving postural control of the head, neck and trunk, improving control of the pharyngeal airway via positioning, normalizing the child's response to stimulation, maintaining tolerance of taste and facilitation of an effective suck and swallow reflex.
- Avoid therapeutic tastes of foods that produce an increase in mucus (milk-based products, grains and some sweets) and move toward safer small tastes of watery liquid/fruit juice thickened as needed.

Nasogastric and Silastic Feeding Tubes

- A silastic (soft) feeding tube is recommended over a standard nasogastric tube. The silastic tube is less irritating and can remain in place several weeks in the nares vs. three to four days with a standard nasogastric tube. Infants generally tolerate an 8 french silastic tube without difficulty.
- Hypersensitivity and hyperirritability can develop around the mouth due to decreased oral exploration if the child is unable to bring hands to mouth or limited due to the presence of the naso/orogastric tube or lack of feeding input due to gastrostomy tube. Provide the child with an appropriate mouthing program to maintain normal sensation in the oral facial area.
- The child can also habituate to the nasogastric tube and may develop reduced pharyngeal sensitivity as a result as well as decreased activation of the gag reflex.
- Placement of the tube through the nasopharynx prevents complete closure of the soft palate, reducing the build up of intra-oral pressure required for efficient sucking and swallowing and if the tube crosses the tongue root the child may have discomfort with swallowing and start to inhibit normal patterns.

When is a Gastrostomy or PEG Tube the Best Option? How should it be Used?

- Gastrostomy is recommended for the child whose patterns are not likely to change rapidly and who may require tube feedings for more than three to six months.
- Gastrostomy reduces negative oral experiences, however, it can result in increased gastroesophageal reflux. If the child is at risk or has a diagnosis of reflux, a GJ tube or jejunostomy may need to be considered.
- The family will be trained in use, cleaning and care of the g-tube prior to the child's discharge from the hospital. Most children remain in the hospital for 24-hours after placement of the tube for instruction time with the family and for the team to make sure the tube is working well. Parents should only use formula, breastmilk or pediasure for the g-tube feedings. Baby foods or pureed foods are not recommended due to decreased osmolarity, risk of clogging the tube and risk of infection due to bacteria in foods that have been reheated or processed.
- The dietitian will recommend a g-tube feeding schedule that best meets the needs of the individual child.

133

Evaluation and Treatment of Pediatric Feeding Disorders: From NICU to Childhood

What about Reflux? Is a Nissen Fundoplication Needed?

Be advised that a Nissen fundoplication may reduce reflux but may result in other problems such as decreased esophageal motility, pain, gastroparesis and dumping syndrome as well as increased aversion. The technique used by the gastroenterologist/surgeon is critical to success of fundoplication. Children with tone issues may not always be good candidates for a fundoplication.

Surgical Management of Reflux: Is a Nissen Fundoplication needed?

"For children with suspective aversive feeding behaviors and without suspected GER, evaluation by a trained speech-language pathologist will determine whether additional diagnostic evaluation for oral or pharyngeal motor dysfunction is warranted before commencing with intensive feeding therapy. If indicated a VFSS (videofluoroscopic swallow study or modified barium swallow study) will determine whether the airway is protected from aspiration, and it will assist the therapist in evaluating swallowing of thick vs. thin liquids.

Primary G-tube placement is performed in children who demonstrate oropharyngeal aspiration. As follow-up of these children suggests, an antireflux procedure at the time or GER diagnosis or G-tube insertion is not necessary, although all children with gastrostomies received acid suppression therapy with H2-receptor antagonists. Oral nutrition supplements alone often are sufficient to achieve nutritional adequacy for patients without evidence of aspiration. For children with a history consistent with GER, including patients with swallowing dysfunction and those with 24-hour pH monitoring, scintigraphy and endoscopy will identify candidates for additional medical therapy or surgery. Fundoplications are absolutely indicated only for patients who manifest reflux-associated aspiration. At present, we recommend antireflux procedures for patients with moderate to severe esophagitis (Hill's grade II-IV).

Additional studies are needed to define the ideal medical therapy for GER, to evaluate responses to nonsurgical treatment after the withdrawl of cisipride from the US market, and to determine whether antireflux procedures ultimately will be needed in patients with GER but without secondary complications."

> --Schwarz S, Corredor J, Fisher-Medina J, Cohen J, Rabinowitz S: Diagnosis and Treatment of Feeding Disorders in Children with Developmental Disabilities. Pediatrics Vol. 108, Number 3, Sept 2001

Transition to Oral Feedings

Premature removal of the tube may lead the child into dehydration or a pattern of failure to thrive. The feeding therapist should rely on the physician/dietitian to direct the transition back to oral feedings. A team approach is needed to successfully achieve oral feeding goals during the transition to oral feedings. The pediatric gastroenterologist, pediatrician or primary physician, dietitian, speech therapist and occupational therapist, home health staff and parents must work together.

Nutrition and Digestive Disorders

When transitioning back to oral feedings, work to improve the rhythmic sucking patterns and establish a foundation of appropriate feeding skills. Make sure skills are appropriate to support full oral feeding.

Parenteral Nutrition

Total or partial parenteral nutrition or PPN/TPN can provide nutritional support to neonates, but may also be used in conjunction with enteral nutrition to provide partial daily requirements for certain infants.

Indications for TPN in the neonatal period include: surgical gastrointestinal disorders such as gastroschisis, tracheoesophageal fistula, malrotation, etc., intractable diarrhea of infancy, short bowel syndrome, NEC, gastrointestinal fistulas, hypermetabolic states, renal failure, cystic fibrosis, cardiac and hepatic failure and sepsis.

Complications are varied from administration of TPN and may include metabolic disturbances, cholestatic jaundice, fatty acid deficiency, hyperlipidemia, dehydration, vitamin inbalance, rickets, infection, and hyper or hypoglycemia.

Disorders and Dysphagia Reference Guide

Dr. Rudolph classified disorders into categories for physicians and feeding team members for a quick reference guide.

DISORDERS THAT AFFECT APPETITE AND INGESTION

Disorders include: depression, deprivation, central nervous system disease, metabolic diseases, sensory defects, neuromuscular disease, oral hypersensitivity or aversion, conditioned dysphagia (aspiration, GER, dumping syndrome), fatigue, poverty and anorexia nervosa.

DISORDERS THAT AFFECT ORAL, PHARYNGEAL AND ESOPHAGEAL SWALLOWING

Disorders include: anatomic abnormalities of the oropharynx (cleft lip or palate, macroglossia, lingual ankyloglossia, Pierre-Robin malformation sequence, cleft larynx, retropharyngeal mass or abcess), anatomic abnormalities of the esophagus (TE fistula, congenital esophageal atresia, congenital esophageal stenosis, esophageal web, stricture or ring, esophageal mass, foreign body or vascular rings), disorders affecting suck/swallow/breathe sequence (CP, bulbar palsy, brain stem glioma, Arnold-Chiari malformation, myelomeningocele, familial dysautonomia, Tardive dyskinesia, Nitrazepam-induced dysphagia, Mobius syndrome, Myasthenia Gravis, infant botulism, congenital myotonic dystrophy, oculopharyngeal dystrophy, muscular dystrophy, cricopharyngeal achalasia, polymyositis/dermatomyosistis and rheumatoid arthritis).

135

DISORDERS AFFECTING ESOPHAGEAL PERISTALSIS

Disorders include: achalasia, Chagas disease, diffuse esophageal spasm, pseudoobstruction, Scleroderma, mixed connective tissue disease, systematic lupus erythematosus, polymyositis/dermatomyositis and rheumatoid arthritis.

MUCOSAL INFECTIONS AND INFLAMMATORY DISORDERS CAUSING DYSPHAGIA

Disorders include: candida pharyngitis or esophagitis, peptic esophagitis, herpes simplex esophagitis, human immunodeficiency virus infection, cytomegalovirus esophagitis, medication-induced esophagitis, Crohn's disease, Behcet disease and chronic graft-versus-host disease.

MISCELLANEOUS DISORDERS ASSOCIATED WITH FEEDING AND SWALLOWING DISORDERS

Disorders include: xerostomia, hypothyroidism, neonatal hyperparathyroidism, trisomy 18 and 21, Prader-Willi syndrome, allergies, lipid and lipoprotein metabolism disorders, neurofibromatosis, Williams syndrome, Coffin-Siris syndrome, Opitz-G syndrome, Cornelia de Lange syndrome, interstitial deletion, globus pharyngeus and epidermolysis bullosa dystrophica.

FAILURE TO THRIVE

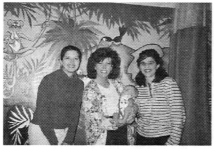

▲ *First Birthday* ▲

This infant with severe failure to thrive, pictured with his therapists, is celebrating his first birthday. This picture demonstrated how some premature infants struggle with failure to thrive after discharge. This diagnosis affects all aspects of a child's development. While making recommendations it is necessary that a therapist formulate a treatment plan specific to that child, despite the child's chronological age, adjusted age, or developmental norms.

Failure to thrive is frequently seen in NICU graduates and described as height, weight and head circumference growth delays.

TYPES OF FAILURE TO THRIVE

Failure to thrive can be classified as organic due to major illness or organ system failure or non-organic due to the child being in a non-nurturing environment or mixed FTT. Many children who have been diagnosed with nonorganic failure to thrive have subtle neuromuscular or oral-motor disorders.

ETIOLOGY

FTT can be caused by CNS damage and related feeding problems, cardio-pulmonary disorders, metabolic disorders, abnormalities of the endocrine system, malabsorption, reflux and chronic gastroenteritis, genetic disorder (such

Nutrition and Digestive Disorders

as Cystic Fibrosis), infections, exposure to parasites and from economic, social and psychological problems.

ASSOCIATED MEDICAL CONDITIONS

Failure to thrive is associated with medical conditions that impact coordination of the suck/swallow/breathe sequence such as:

KRABBE'S DISEASE

A genetic disease only transferred by both the mother and father. It is not determined by gender. The disease does not allow for proper nerve development in the brain. The myelin sheath does not form correctly. The CNS is impacted and seizures can develop. Digestion is inhibited. The disease eventually affects all brain areas and the nerves begin to die. This is a progressive and terminal illness that presents between 2 to 9 months of age. In some cases, there is late onset of symptoms. Early signs include: severe irritability, body or limb rigidity, loss of milestones, severe reflux, feeding trouble, unexplained fevers and unusual eye movements.

TAY-SACHS DISEASE

Tay-Saches disease is a genetic disorder in children that causes progressive destruction of the central nervous system (CNS). Tay-Sachs is terminal. It is caused by an absence of the enzyme hexosaminidase A (Hex-A) and without it, a fatty substance (lipid) called ganglioside accumulates abnormally in the cells, especially the cells of the brain. This ongoing accumulation causes progressive damage to the cells. The destructive process begins in the fetus early in the pregnancy, although the disease is not clinically apparent until the child is several months old. Even with the best of care, all children with classical TSD die early in childhood, usually before age five. Initial symptoms are loss of peripheral vision, abnormal startle response, diminishing mental function, and progressive inability to swallow.

MOBIUS SYNDROME

Mobius Syndrome is incomplete development of the 6th and 7th (accessory and facial) cranial nerves that affects the eyes and muscles of the face. Infants have absent suck, may have abnormalities in development of the tongue, may not be able to blink or move their eyes, can have hearing problems and as well as submucous cleft of the palate.

Treatment of FTT

TEAM ASSESSMENT

FTT requires assessment by an experienced pediatric team including physician/specialists, dietitian, speech therapist, occupational therapist, nursing service, social work service and behavioral psychologist.

Team will assess if the child has normal absorption, hunger patterns, the ability to take enough food by mouth to meet nutritional needs and will determine if there are any problems at home/daycare and with other caregivers that are preventing adequate intake.

MEDICAL EVALUATION AND MEDICATIONS

- The child has a full medical evaluation to determine if there are underlying digestive tract disorders.
- If symptoms of gastroesophageal reflux are significant, the child may have a ph-probe to assess degree of reflux.
- If the physician suspects other disorders, such as eosinophilic gastroenteritis, the child may have a scoping procedure to biopsy the tissue in the esophagus.
- Blood tests may be completed to rule out celiac disease and other disorders.
- The child may also have a sweat test to rule out cystic fibrosis.
- Medications such as Prevacid, Prilosec or Zantac may be prescribed to children with gastroesophageal reflux. Reglan may be prescribed in special cases to improve stomach emptying, however, there are many side effects to consider before prescribing Reglan. Mirilax, Lactulose or Milk of Magnesia may be prescribed to treat constipation problems.

HEIGHT AND WEIGHT CHARTS

- The child's height and weight are plotted by the dietitian. This helps the team determine current status and determine if the child is ready to begin a treatment program.
- The team also looks carefully at the time period when the child first started losing weight. If weight loss occurred after baby food or cow's milk was introduced, allergy testing may be completed.
- As many of these children also exhibit behavioral feeding problems, the child must be ready for the program and be physically able to have the occasional meal or snack with poor intake without jeopardizing health status.
- A child who is too low weight may lose appetite to the point of childhood anorexia and will not respond to the structured meal schedule and may actually lose more ground if treatment is started too early.
- Some children are so underweight that they require caloric supplements (Nutren Jr., Pediasure, Kindercal or NuBasics Juice in rare cases) prior to treatment. Supplements may be given via nasogastric feedings or oral feedings for a few weeks prior to implementation of the feeding program. Weight must be adequate to start a treatment program. Some children will burn too many calories trying to consume caloric supplements orally.
- Slow drip nasogastric feedings for a few weeks will often help the child put on sufficient weight to regain appetite. In most cases, home nursing care will assist the family with the NG feedings as well as monitor weight; however, some children are hospitalized for this stage of treatment.

FOOD LOGS

- Food logs are taken for a three-day period and also analyzed by the dietitian and feeding team members.

Nutrition and Digestive Disorders

- Food logs give the team an idea of when the child eats during the day, the typical volume of foods and liquid and food logs also help the term start setting initial goals via food chaining.
- Many children immediately increase their intake of food if juices, sodas and sugared drinks are eliminated from their diet.

OTHER EVALUATIONS

- If the child demonstrates symptoms of a sensory-based feeding disorder, occupational therapy is consulted to evaluate the child.
- Physical and occupational therapy services may be needed if the child requires a seating system (wheelchair, adaptive equipment) due to motor challenges.
- Mind-Body Medicine/Child Life or Behavioral psychology consults may be needed for children who have experienced a trauma, such as a choking spell.
- Biofeedback therapy often works well for children with a fear of eating.

BEHAVIOR INTERVENTION

- If there are significant behaviors impacting feeding, the team designs a treatment program directed by the behavioral psychologist.
- The family is instructed how to start shaping and extinguishing behaviors prior to implementing the program. If the parent does not maintain consistent response to negative behaviors, the chances of that behavior occurring again increase by 300%.
- All family members must agree to follow the program as written without exception. Extended family members are contacted (when appropriate) and advised of the guidelines of the feeding program.
- Problems are reported to the team leader and modifications are made as needed.
- Behavioral feeding programs are also developed for home, daycare and all feeding situations (birthday parties, family gatherings) to maintain a consistent program.

Gastroesophageal Reflux/Chalasia

Reflux is the spontaneous return of gastric contents into the esophagus.

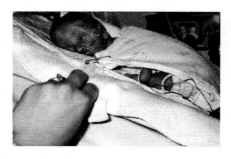

This infant is positioned on a wedge at a 45-degree angle in reflux precautions.

(Photo courtesy of St. John's Hospital, Springfield, Illinois.)

▲ *Baby on wedge* ▲

FEEDING SYMPTOMS

- Baby may feed well initially and then start squirming and writhing within the first 5 minutes of the feeding or he may reject the bottle.
- Reflux is patternless, it can occur five minutes after a feeding or two hours after the feeding is finished.
- May see bradycardic spells (heart rate below 100 bpm) associated with reflux.
- Baby does not have to "spit up" to be a reflux case. Silent reflux may occur.
- Baby may start arching (Note: Arching is also an infant response sign of swallow dysfunction as well as other motoric problems, assess carefully)
- Baby may cough or gag in their crib while sleeping.

IS THERE A PATTERN TO REFLUX OR VOMITING?

Reflux is random and does not follow a pattern. The term "vomiting" is used to describe a more forceful event. Vomiting that occurs regularly or with increased severity may indicate a more significant problem, such as pyloric stenosis,malrotation with midgut volvus or cyclic vomiting syndrome. Pyloric stenosis is usually evident in the first weeks of life.

COMPOLICATED VS. UNCOMPLICATED REFLUX

Reflux is a problem or complicated if it is accompanied by poor weight gain, blue spells, chronic URI/pneumonia and feeding refusals. The health is compromised in some way due to reflux.

Uncomplicated reflux may occur every feeding, but the baby is thriving, healthy and shows no change in health due to reflux. This baby is known as the "happy spitter."

DOES FORMULA CHANGE HELP?

Reflux is mechanical by nature and is not influenced by the type of formula given to the child. Children who do not tolerate formula have a different underlying problem, not pure reflux. Special formulas will help these children.

WHY ARE PREMATURE INFANTS SO PRONE TO REFLUX?

A the premature infant may experience an increased risk to reflux due to respiratory compromise and the resulting imbalance in the pressure gradient between the stomach and the chest.

The lower esophageal sphincter lies in the diaphragm but may be pulled upward slightly in the preemie. LES pressure is lower in the premature infant but the sphincter still serves as a barrier to reflux. The LES relaxes when we swallow.

WHAT ARE SOME OF THE OTHER COMPLICATIONS CAUSED BY REFLUX?

GER can cause reflex laryngospasm, i.e., partial or total closure of the airway. Reflux can also cause pressure on the vagal nerve resulting in bradycardia.

An infant with thrush can develop candida esophagitis (thrush is also present in the esophagus), which can contribute to feeding aversion/refusal.

Reflux may also cause esophagitis and contribute to a future feeding aversion or lead to aspiration of gastric content.

TREATMENT

- Reflux treatment includes positioning management by elevated head of the bed or use of a wedge and Tucker Sling.
- Right sidelying position after feeding for better stomach emptying (may be contraindicated for some cardiac infants).
- Feedings on a schedule with adequate time for stomach emptying; thickened feedings with blenderized rice cereal (1/2 tsp. Per ounce).
- Medications such as Prilosec, Prevacid or Zantac may be prescribed.
- Referral to pediatric gastroenterologist is recommended. Some patients may require diagnostic testing such as, a ph-probe, upper GI with or without small bowel follow through, EGD (scoping procedure with biopsy as needed) and tests for allergies for children with significant history.
- If the child is experiencing complicated reflux, the therapist may need to complete a modified barium swallow/FEES evaluation of the swallow to rule out direct aspiration.
- The therapist may switch baby to a bottle that reduces air intake, such as, the Dr. Brown Bottle with the Level II nipple (medium flow) or Y-cut nipple if using cereal with the feeding. If you use the Dr. Brown Bottle and Y nipple you do not have to blenderize the cereal.
- With high flow nipples, thicken formula with blenderized rice or oatmeal cereal (Beech Nut has finest flakes, blenderize dry cereal in a blender to a powder consistency). We suggest 1/2 tsp per ounce; increase as needed.
- Chalasia precautions (elevated and side-lying positioning, frequent burp breaks with as little movement as possible, wait 5 to 10 minutes to burp final time to allow air bubbles to rise) may help reduce symptoms and provide additional airway protection from gastric content.

SPECIAL CONSIDERATION

- Rib cage treatment, especially in children who are premature or with CNS disorders, may be indicated. The ribcage may be very high in the chest and rib cage treatment can ease symptoms. This form of treatment involves referral to a pediatric physical or occupational therapist.
- There is a balance between the pressure gradient in the chest and the abdomen that needs to be maintained. Premature infants have immature lungs and are very susceptible to reflux as the lower esophageal sphincter is pulled up out of the surrounding diaphragm and pressure gradient is not equal. Reduce mobility secondary to motor delays also inhibits descent of the rib cage as the child develops. (Co-treatment in an aqua therapy program with PT/OT is also a good option.)
- Medical management may be needed if reflux is severe and compromises respiratory function.
- Medical management includes medications or surgical intervention with a *Nissan fundoplication.* A fundoplication is a surgical procedure to tighten the base of the lower esophageal sphincter. This procedure is usually completed when reflux results in aspiration of gastric content. In most cases of

gastroesophageal reflux, other forms of treatment should be explored prior to fundoplication.

- Be advised that fundoplication can also cause problems with gastroparesis (delayed emptying) or dumping syndrome (rapid emptying) and suggest it only after attempting other management strategies or when the child is at great risk for aspiration of gastric content.

Eosinophilic Gastoenteritis

Children are often referred for feeding therapy as they have developed an aversion to eating from the associated epigastric pain and severe vomiting. Eosinophilic gastroenteritis is an infiltrative disorder of the GI tract that affects young children and adults. The condition may be related to an allergic or immunologic reaction, as symptoms tend to follow ingestion of certain foods.

Affected patients tend to have a history of food allergy. In this condition there is extensive infiltration of one or all layers (mucosa, submucosa, muscular) of the stomach and/or small bowel by eosinophils and it can spread to the esophagus or other organs.

SYMPTOMS

The child presents with delayed onset of vomiting starting around 7-8 months of age may be reported in infants as they are reacting to inflammation after baby foods have been added to their diet. Symptoms include epigastric pain, vomiting and diarrhea, bloating and nausea. Patients can also develop a protein losing enteropathy due to increased mucosal permeability, which results in hypoalbuminemia and hypogammaglobulinemia (also causing weight loss).

HOW IS EOSINOPHILIS GASTROENTERITIS DIAGNOSED AND TREATED?

It is diagnosed via biopsy during an EGD (scoping procedure). Treatment consists of steroids and/or removal of sensitizing agent. Young children are fed only with elemental formulas and then foods are gradually re-introduced. Patient should be followed by a pediatric dietitian.

Cyclic Vomiting Syndrome (CVS)

WHAT IS CYCLIC VOMITING SYNDROME?

Cyclic vomiting syndrome is characterized by bouts or cycles of severe nausea and vomiting that last for hours or days and alternates with longer periods of no symptoms.

INCIDENCE

CVS occurs mostly in children (1 in 50 have the disorder), but the disorder can affect adults also.

WHAT ARE THE SYMPTOMS

Attacks tend to start the same time of day, last the same length of time and present at the same level of intensity. However, some children may not follow a clear onset pattern.

Vomiting is sometimes so severe and violent that the patient may vomit or retch 6-10 or up to 50 times per hour, in some cases vomiting is almost constant.

Other symptoms include pallor; exhaustion, listlessness and the patient may almost appear unconscious with extreme sensitivity to light. Headache, fever, dizziness, diarrhea and abdominal pain may also accompany an episode.

Vomiting may cause drooling and excessive thirst. Drinking water may cause more vomiting, however, water can dilute the acid in the vomit, making the episode a little less painful.

ETIOLOGY AND DIAGNOSIS

CVS has no known cause but is associated with abdominal migraine. It can be triggered by stress or excitement or occur with another illness. It is diagnosed by symptoms; there is no known test for CVS. CVS is underdiagnosed and usually identified by a pediatric gastroenterologist or neurologist.

PHASES OF CYCLIC VOMITED ATTACKS

Phases are:
- Prodrome (abdominal pain, onset of nausea, may be a few minutes long or several hours).
- Episode (the attack).
- Recovery (rehydration and electrolyte treatment).
- Symptom-free interval (days, weeks or months).

RISK FACTORS

Risk factors include: severe dehydration and electrolyte imbalance, tooth decay, and peptic esophagitis. Mallory-Weiss tear (lower end of the esophagus may tear open) or the stomach may bruise from vomiting/retching spells.

TREATMENT

There is no definitive treatment for CVS. Medications for migraines Propranolol, Cyproheptadine and Amitriptyline are sometimes used during the prodrome phase (1st), but they do not work for every patient. Many children improve after diagnosis as stress is reduced once the disorder is identified. Symptoms may ease with age or the child may develop migraine headaches.

Treatment involves determining triggers for CVS and trying to decrease the effect on the patient. Relaxation therapy, frequent small meals and medications to aid in healing of the esophagus may also benefit the patient.

Evaluation and Treatment of Pediatric Feeding Disorders: From NICU to Childhood

Pyloric Stenosis

WHAT IS PYLORIC STENOSIS?

The pylorus is a short muscular tube that connects the stomach to the duodenum, the first section of the small intestine. In pyloric stenosis, the muscular wall of the tube thickens and the passageway inside narrows. As a result, little or no milk can pass from the stomach into the intestines and the baby does not get enough nutrients. Pyloric stenosis occurs in 3/1000 births.

WHAT ARE THE SYMPTOMS?

Between 1-10 weeks of age the baby begins to vomit violently after feedings, projectile vomiting is often reported. Because of the narrowing, food is forced up the esophagus with great force.

There is a palpable mass in the epigastric area and during the feeding strong contractions of the stomach may be visible. In some cases, it can resemble a golf ball traveling from left to right beneath the surface of the skin. Emesis is often curdled and contains mucus. The baby wants to eat but will soon lose weight. Results in dehydration and weight loss.

HOW IS PYLORIC STENOSIS TREATED?

Pyloric stenosis is diagnosed by UGI and ultrasound and treated surgically.

Duodenal Atresia and Stenosis

Infants with duodenal atresia may present with vomiting in the first few hours of life. Infants with stenosis present at variable times, depending on the degree of the stenosis. Duodenal atresia and stenosis are a common finding in Down syndrome.

Midgut Volvus

WHAT IS MIDGUT VOLVUS?

This is the most common form of small bowel volvulus. The entire gut twists and spirals around the superior mesenteric artery and vein and the resulting vascular compromise results in necrosis and perforation. If not diagnosed, child can lose significant portion of the small bowel.

WHAT ARE THE SYMPTOMS?

The patient presents with bilious vomiting.

WHAT IS THE TREATMENT FOR MIDGUT VOLVUS?

144

Diagnosed by upper GI, may be difficult to determine on x-ray. Treatment is surgery.

Hirschsprung's Disease

DEFINITION

Hirschsprung's Disease is aganglionosis of the colon. The involved segment does not relax to allow for passage of stool. A baby with Hirschsprungs will not pass a stool without assistance, such as with rectal stimulation and suppositories or an enema.

SYMPTOMS

Typical presentation is vomiting, abdominal distention and failure to pass meconium the first 24-36 hours of life. Commonly involves the distal colonic segment the rectal and rectosigmoid areas. Diagnosed by rectal biopsy.

Malabsorption

DEFINITION

Malabsorption results from structural changes in the small intestine or if chemicals and enzymes within the small intestine are not properly assisting the digestive process.

ASSOCIATED DISORDERS

Associated with Celiac disease, Crohn's disease, lactase deficiency, iron-deficiency anemia, B12 anemia, pancreatitis, diabetes mellitus, cystic fibrosis (the pancreas does not produce any enzymes or digestive juices to break down food) and can occur after digestive tract surgery.

SYMPTOMS

Symptoms include abdominal discomfort, loose bowels, yellow-gray, greasy looking bowel movements that have a particularly strong odor and tend to float due to high fat content.

COMPLICATIONS

Untreated leads to weight loss, lethargy and the symptoms of vitamin deficiency begin including sore tongue, prickling sensation and numbness in the arms and legs, bone pain, muscle cramps.

HOW IS MALABSORPTION DIAGNOSED AND TREATED?

It is diagnosed by a blood test and stool sample, and is treated with a high protein, high calorie diet and vitamin/mineral supplements.

Celiac Disease

DEFINITION

Celiac disease is an allergy that affects the small intestine and is one of the most common malabsorption disorders.

WHAT HAPPENS IN THE INTESTINAL TRACT?

Gluten, a product in most grains, comes in contact with the membrane that lines the small intestine and causes blunting of the villi. This loss of villi and resulting smooth lining of the intestine reduces the normal absorption of nutrients.

WHAT ARE THE SYMPTOMS

Symptoms begin after cereals are introduced in the diet, and include the following: weight loss or slow gain, poor appetite, loose, pale, foul smelling bowel movements, gas, distended abdomen, ulcers in the mouth, anemia and vitamin deficiency.

HOW IS CELIAC DISEASE DIAGNOSED AND TREATED?

Celiac Disease is diagnosed via blood tests and/or biopsy of the lining of the intestine, and treatment involves removing gluten from the diet. Rice and corn are safe to eat. The child will need special gluten free breads and a gluten free diet for life. Patient will need to be followed by a pediatric dietitian.

Lactose Intolerance

WHAT IS LACTOSE INTOLERANCE?

Lactase is produced in the lining of the small intestine and breaks down lactose, the sugar in cow's milk. True lactose intolerance is actually quite rare. Reduction in the amount of lactase can cause intolerance and digestive problems with milk products.

WHAT ARE THE SYMPTOMS

If present at birth it causes bloating and persistent diarrhea immediately and baby does not gain weight.

WHAT ARE THE COMPLICATIONS OF LACTOSE INTOLERANCE?

Severe gastroenteritis in a baby can temporarily damage the lining of the intestine and reduce or cease lactase production resulting in diarrhea and vomiting. Possibility of failure to thrive.

TREATMENT

The child is placed on special lactose free formulas and milk may gradually re-introduced.

Ulcerative Colitis

WHAT IS ULCERATIVE COLITIS?

An inflammatory bowel diseases resulting in inflammation and sores, ulceration that forms in the top layers of the lining of the large intestine. Inflammation usually occurs in the rectum and lower section of the colon; however, it may also affect the entire colon.

Ulcerative colitis rarely affects the small intestine, except for the ileum and damage is deeper within the intestinal wall than with Crohn's disease. The patient has abnormalities of the immune system, but it is not known is this is a cause or symptom of the disease.

WHO IS PRONE TO ULCERATIVE COLITIS?

Ulcerative Colitis usually occurs between the ages of 15 to 40 years of age, but can occur in children and the elderly. Patients often have stress and/or depression trying to cope with these inflammatory disorders. Teenage patients are particularly stressed by these challenges.

WHAT ARE THE SYMPTOMS OF ULCERATIVE COLITIS?

Symptoms include fatigue, weight loss, loss of appetite, rectal bleeding, loss of body fluids and nutrients. Other more severe problems are frequent fever, bloody diarrhea, nausea, severe abdominal cramps, liver disease, osteoporosis, skin rashes, anemia, kidney stones, inflammation of the eyes and arthritis.

HOW IS ULCERATIVE COLITIS DIAGNOSED AND TREATED?

- Diagnosed via colonoscopy and barium enema may be required.
- Treatment is with medications such as corticosteroids and 5-ASA agents (Sulfasalazine) diet change or surgery to remove diseased sections of the colon.
- Nutritional support may be needed.
- Stress counseling (from dealing with the disorder) and relaxation therapy may benefit the patient. UC and CD are not stress-related disorders, however they lead to symptoms of stress or depression in many patients.
- Surgery is the only cure and several types are done. Proctocolectomy with ileostomy is one of the most common surgeries. The surgeon removes the colon and rectum and creates a stoma in the abdomen for waste to exit the body.
- There are special support groups and camps for children with ulcerative colitis.

Evaluation and Treatment of Pediatric Feeding Disorders: From NICU to Childhood

WHAT ARE THE COMPLICATIONS OF THIS DISEASE?

Complications include severe illness, rupture of the colon, massive bleeding and the risk of colon cancer.

Crohn's Disease

WHAT IS CROHN'S DISEASE?

Crohn's disease is the second of the inflammatory bowel diseases that damages the wall of the gastrointestinal tract. CD usually occurs between the ages of 15-40 and is characterized by periods of inflammation and followed by periods of remission. Women are affected 20% more often than men and the disease has a familial component.

The disease usually occurs in the small intestine, but can be found in the mouth, esophagus, stomach, duodenum, large intestine, appendix and anus. Scarring from damage to the tract can lead to malabsorption.

WHAT ARE THE SYMPTOMS OF CROHN'S DISEASE?

Symptoms include periodic attacks of cramps, lower right abdominal pain, diarrhea, general feeling of ill health and slight fever. If continues for years causes gradual deterioration of bowel functioning. There is a higher risk of anemia, malabsorption, weight loss and peritonitis.

HOW IS CROHN'S DISEASE TREATED?

Medical treatment focuses on minimizing symptoms and complications, improving nutrition, moving the patient into a remission stage with drug treatment to control inflammation and to avoid surgery.

Dumping Syndrome

WHAT IS DUMPING SYNDROME?

Dumping Syndrome usually caused by certain types of stomach surgery that allows the stomach to empty rapidly. Dumping syndrome can occur after a Nissen fundoplication. After surgery, patients can develop abdominal bloating, pain, vomiting, vasomotor symptoms (flushing, sweating, lightheadedness, diarrhea) as fluid from the blood moves to the dilute intestinal contents. This "early" phase of dumping syndrome may occur 30-60 minutes after eating, "late phase" dumping occurs approximately two hours after eating as a result of low blood sugars. Under normal conditions the stomach and the pylorus control the rate at which gastric contents leave the stomach.

HOW IS DUMPING SYNDROME TREATED?

Patient should be seen by a pediatric gastroenterologist and dietitian to modify treat and to modify the diet and schedule intake of foods and liquids.

148

Additional Resources

CHAPTER ELEVEN

▲

Additional Resources

Comparison of Disposable and Market Brand Nipples
(Fraker and Walbert)

Most normal newborn infants can feed well with any type of nipple on the market. There are many good products on this chart. If an infant is feeding well in a timely manner with good activation of the musculature, we suggest that you stay with the product that is working for that child. Basically, "if it ain't broke, don't fix it" applies to this patient. However, if the child is feeding and presenting with oral spillage, poor lip seal, arching, fatigue and/or is constantly pulling away from the nipple, a change in the product used may significantly decrease these problems. Nipples vary dramatically in texture, size and flow rate. The flow rate may be too fast or the child may need a nipple that is larger in diameter to seal the mouth more effectively or one that is slightly longer to give additional input to the tongue to encourage tongue grooving and facilitate improved bolus control. The purpose of this comparison is to help the therapist match the right nipple to meet the patient's needs. This comparison also provides suggestions for the best products to reduce air intake while feeding for infants, preemie and newborn, with symptoms of colic as well as infants with special needs such as cleft lip and palate.

The "RP rating" (RP = Recommended Product) suggests nipples to use in treatment that specifically work the oral-facial musculature and encourage the development of appropriate feeding skills. The "RP" rating means only that we frequently use the product with our patients due to the fact that it specifically meets the requirements for special needs infants. The therapist should use this comparison chart to select nipples that make the feeding therapeutic and actually exercise the oral facial musculature every time the infant feeds.

This comparison was also completed to give parents of premature infants or infants with special feeding problems the best products to work the oral facial musculature, yet allow adequate intake after they are discharged from the NICU or the hospital. We tried to identify nipples that were the closest to the Ross disposable yellow standard nipple used to feed NICU infants in most hospitals.

149

1. HOSPITAL DISPOSABLE NIPPLES

Ross Red Preemie Ross Blue and Pink Nipples	Compression type nipple, encourages jaw excursion, fast flow rate, designed to take work out of sucking but may increase work at pharyngeal stage of swallowing. Pinks and blues are very small. May work with some infants, but also not recommended as best option. May consider Gerber Preemie Nurser instead. (See info in Special Feeding Systems)	Does not work lips or cheeks effectively, does not facilitate bolus formulation and control. Liquid likely to spill into the cheeks. No comparable nipple available after discharge. Not recommended for long term use. Disposable nipples, will not maintain a constant flow rate or texture with long-term use. Difficult to order for use after discharge. Refer to research study by Lan, et al regarding high flow and slower flow nipples in the NICU.
Ross Yellow Standard Nipple	Slightly rubbery texture, slow to medium flow, slightly longer than the Munchkin nipples, good proprioceptive input provided to tongue, easy to collapse during feeding.	Milk continues to flow when baby pauses to breathe. Recommended nipple for majority of infants in the NICU. Not recommended after discharge due to expense and difficulty with ordering. Disposable nipple, not appropriate for long-term use.
Ross Orthodontic Nipple or Similac Orthodontic Nipple	Fast flow, broad tip, provides good proprioceptive input to mouth. Not typically recommended for preemies due to flow rate, but can work very well with thickened feedings, but product is not always easily available to families after discharge. Works very well on the cleft palate nurser for infants with cleft lip and palate. Must order through Ross company.	No comparable orthodontic nipple on the market. Ross nipple has one hole at the tip and all the other orthodontics have a hole on the top or a hole at the tip and on top. Can be higher cost due to need to order by the case. Good product for thickened feeds and cleft palate babies, but not available except through the hospital or direct order through Ross. Social work may be able to assist the patient's family with ordering.

Additional Resources

2. SLOW-MEDIUM FLOW RATE NIPPLES; OPTIONS FOR TRANSITION FROM THE ROSS YELLOW STANDARD NIPPLE

Often premature infants are sent home from the NICU with no recommendations for nipples to use after discharge. Many parents use a variety of different nipples or cut a nipple to allow their baby to take a sufficient amount of breastmilk or formula. Generally speaking, you are looking for a medium flow nipple that is pliable enough to seal the mouth well, yet firm enough to give input to the tongue to encourage grooving for improved bolus control and that will have enough resistance to activate the lip/cheek musculature. Lip and cheek activation and tongue cupping is vital to the next step in feeding, which is the transition to spoon-feeding. If the child cannot control a liquid bolus well or is receiving therapeutic feedings, a slow flow nipple may be your best option. If you are uncertain about the flow rate and infants ability to swallow, recommend a modified barium swallow and assess thoroughly.

If colic is a complaint, consider changing the infant to the Dr. Brown Bottle Standard and Level II or Y-cut nipple with cereal if ordered. Have the baby feed consistently on this product for 36-48 hours and see if symptoms are decreased.

RP Gerber Silicone Slow Flow Standard Nipple	Excellent proprioceptive input to tongue and palate, firm, consistent flow rate. Does not flow when baby pauses to breathe.	Good, easy to find product with three flow rates. Silicone is recommended over latex style nipple. Less expense to family than ordering disposables from Ross. Works cheeks and lips.
RP Gerber Silicone Medium Flow Standard Nipple	Excellent proprioceptive input to the tongue and palate. Does continue to flow when baby pauses to breathe.	Slightly faster than the Ross Yellow and can be used without thickening with well coordinated infant. Premature infant may need external pacing by the feeder at first. Works cheeks and lips well.
RP Gerber Silicone Fast Flow Standard Nipple	Same as above. Works well with thickened feedings; we compared this product using 1/2 -1 tsp. blenderized cereal. If thickened, does not flow when baby pauses to breathe.	Not recommended without thickening for preemies. Nice for older babies 6-18 months. Works cheeks and lips. We often use this nipple for infants who need thickened feedings due to GER.
Gerber Standard (Yellow)	Medium Flow rate, excellent proprioceptive input to tongue and palate. Slightly oily to touch but nice texture in the mouth. Doesn't collapse during feeding. Slight flowing during pauses.	Has a three-hole design. Very nice product, good option for baby fed with Ross yellow. Works cheeks and lips. May prefer silicone option for NICU infants due history of higher latex exposure.

151

Gerber 3 Hole Nipple (Yellow)	Medium to Fast Flow. Holes are slightly larger than the Gerber standard. Excellent input and does not collapse during feeding. Slight flowing during pauses.	Works the cheeks and lips and helps facilitate a stable jaw during feeding. May need thickened feeding with younger baby.
Healthflow Standard Nipple and Playtex Standard Nipple	Very thin silicone, easily collapsed by the baby. Risk of increased air intake as baby compresses it and keeps sucking air around nipple.	Too soft to work the cheeks and lips for infants with muscle weakness.
RP Dr. Brown Bottle This bottle won the 2000 Gold Medal Excellence in Medical Design award. Physician from Mt. Zion, Illinois who originally developed this system for his child who had severe GER. This bottle is extremely effective in reducing colic symptoms and decreasing spitting. The Dr. Brown Bottle has a patented internal vent system that separates air from liquid during feeding. May be more expensive than traditional bottles, but may well be worth the cost. Contact hospital social work for assistance for families with special financial needs.	Unique positive pressure patented design removes air from feedings. Excellent proprioceptive input, silicone nipple with slow flow, medium flow still has a little resistance to it with the Level II nipple. Good for infants who need a slower flowing medium rate. No vacuum is created and this allows the infant to feed at its own pace. Y-cut flows fast for cereal/formula feedings, design allows for optimal bolus control. Great for infant's with GI distress during feedings or for any infant. Now available in slow, medium and fast flow, standard and wide mouth design.	Works the cheeks and lips and helps facilitate a stable jaw during feeding. Available in two sizes and currently at Infant specialty stores, Wal-Mart and Infants R Us. Internet ordering also available at Handi-Craft.com or 1-800-778-9001. Excellent customer service. Level I slow nipple comes with the bottle when purchased. Replacement Level II is a medium flow nipple and works very well with most infants, preemies or newborns. Y-Cut nipple is made for cereal. We do not blenderize the cereal when using the Y-Cut nipple. We used 1/2 tsp. per ounce for this comparison. Y-Cut nipple can also work for infants with Cleft Palate (see special topics section). Assess the swallow carefully.
Avent Naturally Feeding Bottle Available in a variety of flow rates RP	Silicone nipple, excellent proprioceptive input to lips, tongue and palate. Does not flow during pauses.	May work well with breastfed babies. Also carry a nice line of soft spout cups for transition to cup drinking.
Evenflo Standard Evenflo Cross-Cut for Juice	Thicker texture, rubbery feel and taste. Cross-cut shoots milk to the pharynx. Due to increased risk of premature spillage into the pharynx this product is not recommended for preemies even with thickened feeds.	Standard continues to flow during pauses.

Evenflo Classic Sensitive Response (silicone)	Much better than standard nipple. Narrow tip to nipple. Nice texture. Medium flow. Works well with the infant who compresses the nipple flat while feeding.	Baby must have good lip seal due to narrow nipple. Works the cheeks and lips. Not for a baby with weak musculature. Flows during pauses. A good product for infant with tight tongue to palate position while feeding.
Parents Choice 0+ (Wal Mart) Recommendation: *Good product line for specific patients with reduced lip seal or excessive air intake with feeding	Medium flow, wide tip to nipple. Soft silicone could collapse if baby sucks vigorously. Nice texture, medium flow.	Flows during pauses. Works the cheek musculature. Economically an advantage as there are six nipples per package. Nice for babies with reduced lip seal or excessive air intake with feedings.
Parents Choice 6 months+	Medium fast flow. Same as above. Could use with blenderized rice cereal (1/4 tsp. Per ounce) if increasing caloric density of formula.	Flows rapidly during pauses. Seals the mouth well.
Parents Choice Nuby 0+	Claims to double as a teether. It has bumps over base of nipple. Does not work as a teether, but the nipple is broad and seals well. Med-fast flow.	May bother a sensitive baby. Very nice texture except for nubby area. Seals mouth well.

3. PLAYTEX NURSER STYLE SYSTEMS

This product design works for most typically developing infants; however, in our comparison these nurser style systems do not work the cheek musculature as actively as standard design nipples. Infants with poor lip seal and weak musculature may start a munching pattern of feeding using these products. Cheek musculature may appear shiny and thick at 6-7 months of age in the preemie population if a munching pattern of intake persists over time. Try to break up these patterns to encourage activation of the cheeks to assist in the transition to spoon and cup skills. These products work well for infants who feed better with increased proprioceptive input to the peri-oral region while feeding.

RP HealthFlow Nipples by Johnson and Johnson. Available in Stage 1 or 2.	Excellent product. Stage 1 does not flow during pauses but Stage 2 nipple does flow.	Could be used with feeding thickened with blenderized rice cereal. Good product, works the cheeks and lips and remains stable in the mouth.
Playtex Round Tip Silicone Nipple (0-12 months) Playtex Flat Tip Silicone (0-12 months)	Medium flow rate. Took a long time to get milk flowing and in our comparison noted inconsistent volume per suck. Occasional bursts of formula, not always a stable flow rate. Does not provide proprioceptive input at the level of the other products.	Nipple moves in and out of mouth during sucking, noted frequent breaks in lip seal. Requires lip strength. Could fatigue a preemie. Continues to flow during pauses in feeding. Very little cheek activation during sucking.
Evenflo (all ages)	Medium to fast flow. Preferred over Playtex style, but not at the level of Healthflow Playtex style nipple.	Works the cheeks. Continues to flow during pauses.
Gerber New Traditions Bottle and Interchangable Nipple System	Note: Does not have disposable liners. Good nipple for medium flow rate when purchased as a unit. Fast flow and slow flow replacements are available. Three different styles of nipples available. Recommend the classic and wide mouth dome over the flex style for infants with reduced lip seal.	Can encourage munching pattern as nipple is soft, slick and very pliable. Mild activation of the cheeks during sucking. Again requires lip strength and seal. Noted possible increase in air intake with flex style and continued flow during pauses in feeding with all three styles.
Playtex Precision Flow Wide Shaped Nipple (Available in stages for age and flow rate)	Very similar features to the Gerber New Traditions Nipple. Gerber nipple is a little firmer than Playtex.	Can encourage munching pattern, only mildly works the cheeks. Requires lip strength and seal. Continues to flow during pauses.
Maws Anti-Colic Variflow Nipple	Cross-cut design with medium fast flow. Could be used with blenderized cereal. Claim to have clinical studies that reduce crying. Very similar features to Gerber and Playtex style nipples.	Did not note any difference in this product with others in our comparison. Lightly works the cheek musculature. Requires good lip strength. Flows during pauses in sucking.

Additional Resources

IV. CLEFT PALATE, SPECIAL AND PREEMIE FEEDING SYSTEMS

RP Pigeon Nipple Available from Children's Medical Ventures 1-800-377-3449 For Cleft Palate	Unique design of ½ firm and ½ soft nipple with a valve to reduce air intake. Excellent product. Can be used with or without a squeeze bottle. Can order the pigeon bottle and control the flow rate of the nipple. Higher cost due to special features.	This product and the Dr. Brown Y-cut nipple/bottle are the products we most frequently recommend for feeding cleft palate babies. Available to parents by phoning 800# or on the internet.
Haberman Feeders Preemie, Newborn and Soft Cup	Nice product, but difficult to assemble, some parents feel it doesn't look like a real bottle. Three flow rates. Higher cost due to the special features of the product.	Does not provide the same input or ease of flow that the pigeon nipple does. Tends to come out in bursts back in the pharynx. Check flow rate carefully. Soft cup feeder- good product, but be aware of increased risk of aspiration if not a trained feeder. Train all feeders who will use the product with the infant.
Cleft Palate Nurser	Nipple is long; baby may have difficulty forming a bolus. Liquid may fall prematurely into the pharynx. Reduced proprioceptive input, grainy texture. Irregular bolus size from inconsistent force of squeezing should be addressed in training the feeder.	Not typically recommended with the nipple that comes with the product. Replace the nipple and the product works very well.
Gerber Preemie Bottle	Has a small standard nipple similar in size to the pink preemie nipple. Good proprioceptive input. Slow-medium flow.	Appropriate only for a short time after discharge. Change as the infant grows.
RP for therapy Munchkin Medicator Cup	Must change the nipple to Gerber slow or medium flow. Nipple is designed to give meds and hole is very large. Excellent product for giving medication.	Small bottle (10cc) is nice if you want to do therapeutic taste and limit the amount possible to give the baby.
RP for therapy Hazelbaker FingerFeeder	Hand-held squeeze silicone bulb and tubing to tape on finger of feeder. Good for single bolus swallow practice or to work on tongue positioning/tolerance of liquid in the mouth.	Medela product in the Haberman feeder line.

155

Evaluation and Treatment of Pediatric Feeding Disorders: From NICU to Childhood

ORDERING INFORMATION

Haberman and Hazelbaker FingerFeeder
Products are available through Medela, Inc.
P.O. Box 660, McHenry, IL USA 60051-0660
Phone: 800-435-8316 or 815-363-1166 or Fax 815-363-1246

Dr. Brown Feeding Systems
Available at Wal-Mart and specialty infant stores. Handi-Craft.com will help you locate a store closest to you or to order on-line; excellent customer service.
Phone: 1-800-778-9001

Cleft Palate Nipple System
(Pigeon) Children's Medical Ventures, Inc.; excellent customer service.
Phone: 1-800-377-3449

Gerber, Evenflo, HealthFlow and Playtex products are available at stores throughout the United States. Avent America, Inc., 1-800-542-8368.

General Feeder Instructions Prior to Starting a Behavioral Feeding Program

Parents should read these guidelines carefully and completely before starting a feeding program. Start a program when your child is in good health and feeling fine. Make sure all family members know that the next few days will be very challenging, but should make significant changes at mealtimes. The goals of a feeding program are to stimulate appetite and shape meals into a schedule that encourages good intake throughout the day. Your therapist will be asking you to change the way you have approached mealtime with your child and will help you to identify the behaviors that are negatively impacting feeding. Many times certain patterns of eating or drinking can decrease a child's appetite and as a result the child falls into habits that are rigid, unhealthy and that result in either weight loss or excessive weight gain. The dietitian will be discussing healthy foods for your child and will help you determine the appropriate amount of food and liquid your child needs each day.

We will help your child expand the types of food he can eat and/or identify foods that he can eat safely. The team will identify behaviors that we want to increase and behaviors that we want to extinguish. The only way to do that is for everyone involved to act exactly the same way with your child at every meal. If your child refuses to eat or tantrums, go into "robot mode" and show no response to the behavior. Continue to eat your meal and do not make eye contact or any response to the behavior. Any attention to the behavior only encourages it to happen again. If your child has a good meal, praise him enthusiastically so he knows that he has done something you approve of and he receives the reward of your attention and special privileges. We will also work with and encourage all caregivers, including extended family and daycare providers/school personnel to follow the program after discharge.

The following are recommendations that should be followed for each meal and snack, without exception:

156

Additional Resources

1. We encourage a set schedule of intake for three meals and two-three snacks per day. Meals should last no longer than 30 minutes and snacks should be 10-15 minutes. There should be no additional feedings between scheduled meals and snacks. Nibbling on food in small amounts during the day is called "grazing" and this pattern of intake prevents your child from feeling hungry and often results in the child taking only a few bites of food at meals. A child who is not hungry is going to fight your attempts to feed him. At the end of a day of grazing, your child has not taken a significant volume of food. Many negative behaviors can also come out of a grazing pattern.

2. Drinks such as soda, juice and tea are not recommended for children as these are basically empty calories and can decrease appetite for food. Children should not be given a cup or bottle to carry with them and sip from during the day. Milk should be offered at milk and snack times only. The child can have water between scheduled meals and snacks. We are trying to build internal motivation (hunger) to prompt your child to eat. If your child is on a caloric supplement, such as KinderCal or Pediasure, we will stop the supplement during this intensive stage of treatment in attempt to help your child learn to eat a wider variety or increased amount of food.

3. Praise all positive behaviors. You won't be doing this forever, but you are teaching your child at this stage in treatment. You won't always have to be a "cheerleader" for your child at mealtime; right now you are shaping a desired behavior and teaching your child to do something that will help him grow to be strong and healthy. Ignore negative behaviors completely. Ignore crying, gagging (if not a sign of oral motor dysfunction or swallowing disorder), dropping food, throwing food and other behaviors that you wish to extinguish. Your child wants your attention and will take positive or negative attention from you and still crave more. Ignoring a behavior completely is the way to make it stop occurring.

4. Do not push a feeding too far especially if the child has been eating well. Children do not eat large amounts of food and you can actually be punishing the child for a good meal if you make the mealtime last longer than necessary. If the child eats well in 10 minutes, the meal is over. Praise your child and give him your attention. Your child can sit in the high chair while you finish your meal and play with a toy or just interact with the family. Thirty minutes is the maximum time your child should spend at the table but this does not mean that you make your child eat for thirty minutes.

5. If your child refuses to eat at a meal after two attempts to offer food, the meal is over. Remove the plate from the high chair. Your child may not be hungry at that meal, but you do not want to "short order cook" by offering something else. Your child is controlling you when you immediately go finding something else to please him. If the meal is balanced and appropriate there should be something he will like enough to eat. Your child will also eat more at the next feeding time because he will be hungry. Stay with the plan and on schedule. Your child can play quietly in the high chair but will not be "rewarded" for avoiding a meal by watching television or playing in the playroom.

157

Evaluation and Treatment of Pediatric Feeding Disorders: From NICU to Childhood

6. *If your child refuses to eat and is upset or screaming, ignore the behavior.* This is the time to go into "robot mode." Your child will not be harmed by the behavioral outburst and is safe in the high chair. Every instinct you have will tell you to go to your child. Stop that impulse and remember you are doing what your child needs. Quietly remove the plate from the high chair, do not offer additional food or drinks. Wait it out and do not respond in any way to the behavior, no eye contact or comments. This is how you make this behavior stop occurring. This is the hardest part of the program. If you are not consistent you have increased the chances of the negative behavior occurring again and again by 300%. If you feel you are about to give in, leave the room for a minute and come back. You may also turn the high chair away from the table while the outburst is occurring. Eventually with no response your child will either tire out or stop crying. If you give in, he will cry longer the next time because he has learned that eventually he will get his way.

7. Your child can only have water between meals and snacks. Meals and snacks are scheduled close enough that if the child refuses to eat it won't be too long before they have the opportunity to eat again, yet the meals are scheduled far enough apart to allow for digestion of food and to stimulate appetite. A sample of our schedule is as follows:

    Breakfast: 7:00 AM
    Snack: 9:30 AM
    Lunch: 11:30 AM
    Nap: 12:00-2:00 PM (if age appropriate)
    Snack: 2:30 PM
    Dinner: 5:30 PM
    Snack: 7:30 PM

8. Your child should remain in the high chair for meal/snack time. You are teaching him to spend adequate time at the table. Control the environment in regard to distractions. The television should be turned off, but soft music is fine. If needed, the occupational therapist will discuss appropriate positioning for your child during meals.

9. Make sure portion sizes are age appropriate. Offer balanced meals with choices of a variety of foods. Your child may like foods that you do not. Provide a small amount of the "comfort foods" your child is used to eating along with foods from all the food groups.

10. Eat with your child whenever possible. You want to set up a normal meal environment. As we work your child through the treatment program we will later recommend no short order cooking. Again for your child, this is a matter of choices and consequences. Your child should eat what you prepare for the family. Our team will work with you and your family to help you make this program work for you at home.

Additional Resources

Evaluation of Feeding Skills: Infant/Child

Name_____DOB_____DOS_____

Parent's Names_____#Siblings_____

Other Caregivers_____

Referring Physician_____

Diagnosis_____

Pre-Feeding Observations

Respiration
- ❏ Clear
- ❏ Stridor
- ❏ Labored Breathing
- ❏ Poor secretion management
- ❏ Supplemental Oxygen
- ❏ Tracheotomy: Size_____Type_____
- ❏ Passy-Muir Valve

Communication
- ❏ Non-Verbal
- ❏ Vocalizes
- ❏ Verbal
- ❏ Augmentative Communication Device
- ❏ Sign/Picture System

State: _____
_____
_____
_____
_____

Positioning for Feeding: _____
_____
_____
_____
_____

Feeders and Settings: _____
_____
_____
_____

Structural Observations

Describe:
Lips _____
Teeth _____
Velum _____
Palate _____
Cheeks _____
Mandible _____
Oral Facial Tone _____

Evaluation and Treatment of Pediatric Feeding Disorders: From NICU to Childhood

Page 2 • Evaluation of Feeding Skills: Infant/Child

Oral Peripheral Examination: _____
_____
_____
_____
_____

Oral Reflexes

Describe:
   Root _____
   Suck _____
   Gag _____
   Swallow _____
   Cough _____
   Phasic Bite _____
   Transverse Tongue _____

Feeding Skills

Bottle Feeding: _____
_____
_____
_____
_____

Nipple Used _____*Recommended Nipple* _____

Spoon Feeding Skills: _____
_____
_____
_____
_____

Type of Spoon _____*Recommended Spoon*_____

Cup Drinking: _____
_____
_____
_____
_____

Type of Cup _____*Recommended Cup*_____

Mastication _____
_____
_____
_____
_____

Length of meal: _____
_____

160

Additional Resources

Page 3 • Evaluation of Feeding Skills: Infant/Child

Feeding Interventions Results _____
_____
_____
_____
_____

Initial Treatment Plan _____
_____
_____
_____
_____
_____
_____

Summary _____
_____
_____
_____
_____
_____
_____

Signature   *Date*

Evaluation and Treatment of Pediatric Feeding Disorders: From NICU to Childhood

Fraker-Walbert Feeding History & Referral Guide

I. Patient Information

Name_____DOB_____DOS_____

Parent's Names_____#Siblings_____

Other Caregivers_____

Referring Physician_____ Phone_____

Daycare_____ School_____

Phone_____ Teacher/Sitter_____

II. Medical Information

*Prenatal/medical history, illness and/or current health status, surgeries, allergies or other concerns, and specialists working with the patient:*_____

_____
_____
_____
_____
_____
_____
_____
_____
_____
_____
_____
_____
_____
_____
_____
_____

*Describe a typical day regarding your child's eating behaviors:*_____

_____
_____
_____
_____
_____

Other than parents, who else feeds your child, how frequently and in what setting? When others feed your child, what happens? _____

_____
_____
_____

(Technique for feeding varies feeder to feeder. Investigate positioning strategies used for feeding, utensils, bottle/cup used, mealtime environment and the feeding schedule. Are the feeders consistent?)

Additional Resources

Page 2 • Fraker-Walbert Feeding History and Referral Guide

Concerns? Do you want us to work with other family members or caregivers to help them follow a consistent feeding technique? _____
_____
_____
_____
_____

III. Feeding Schedule

How often does your infant/child like to eat or drink? Typical intake hourly: _____
_____
_____
_____
_____

AM								PM													AM			
5	6	7	8	9	10	11	12	1	2	3	4	5	6	7	8	9	10	11	12	1	2	3	4

(Grazing patterns will reduce intake and dampen appetite. Suggest structured meals and snacks.)

How many ounces of liquid does your child take during a 24-hour period? _____
_____
(Children with low fluid intake may also have problems with constipation and this can lead to reduced oral intake of foods.)

How long does it take for your child to:
   Breastfeed _____   Drink from a cup _____
   Bottle feed _____   Finish a meal _____
(Meals that exceed thirty minutes result in high calorie burning patterns that may result in poor weight gain; may also indicate oral motor/positioning problems that impact feeding efficiency.)

IV. Positioning

What position does your child prefer to be in during feeding? _____
_____
_____
_____
_____
_____

(Appropriate positioning is vital to successful feeding. Placing infants in car seats or swings can increase problems with reflux due to increased pressure on the abdominal region. Make sure the baby is adequately positioned with an extended ribcage and with reduced abdominal pressure. If the baby is difficult to position or appears to have tone problems, refer to occupational or physical therapy for assistance. Breastfeeding infants also have special positioning needs. For assistance, contact a lactation consultant or OT/PT.)

V. The Breastfed Infant

How frequently does your baby want to nurse? _____
_____
_____
_____

Evaluation and Treatment of Pediatric Feeding Disorders: From NICU to Childhood

Page 3 • Fraker-Walbert Feeding History and Referral Guide

(Infants go through periodic growth spurts and breastfeed very frequently. Many times the mother feels she isn't giving her baby enough milk because of the increased frequency of nursing, when in fact the baby is going through a normal stage of development.)

Any problems with milk supply? _____

_____

(How frequently is the mother pumping? Is her nutrition and fluid intake adequate? If she is hyperlactating she may need to alter her feeding method. Refer to lactation specialist for any problems with milk supply or latch-on.)

How many wet/soiled diapers per day? _____

_____

How does your infant act while feeding? _____

_____

_____

(Pulling away, choking, coughing, arching are red flags. Refer to a feeding specialist and a lactation consultant.)

Have you ever been seen by a lactation consultant? _____

_____

_____

_____

VI. The Bottle-Fed Infant

What formula is your child taking at this time? _____

_____

_____

_____

*Have you used other brands of formula?*_____

_____

_____

("Formula Roulette" is common in infants with reflux or colic. Explore the symptoms the baby presents with before, during and after feeding. Check lip seal and the nipple used and consider changing to a bottle that reduces air intake. Report symptoms to the physician and dietitian for guidance regarding use of an appropriate formula.)

Have you noticed any difference? _____

_____

_____

_____

Have you tried baby food yet? How does your child respond? Any problems? _____

_____

_____

_____

(Reflux or vomiting that increases in severity after baby food is introduced is a red flag. Contact the physician, dietitian and/or pediatric gastroenterologist.)

Additional Resources

Page 4 • Fraker-Walbert Feeding History and Referral Guide

VII. Child Section

*Do you feel your child likes to eat?*_____

_____

_____

_____

(Children refuse foods for a reason. Investigate safety of the swallow and the mealtime environment, appetite and pattern of intake during the day. A child who has little or no interest in eating may be taking small amounts of liquids throughout the day or nibbling on snacks dampening appetite. Try scheduled intake of foods and liquids and offer water only between feedings. No appetite and a child who appears lethargic/weak/pale should be reported to the physician immediately.)

What are your child's favorite foods/drinks? _____

_____

_____

_____

(Are favorite foods all in the same flavor/texture family?)

Are any food/liquids difficult for your child to eat/drink?

_____

_____

_____

_____

(May indicate need for oral motor/feeding therapy. Refer to speech pathology.)

Is your child drinking from a cup? What type? Did your child transition well to cup drinking? Does your child like to carry the sip cup around while he plays?

_____

_____

_____

_____

_____

(If the child is having difficulty transitioning to cup, carefully assess the swallow and oral motor function. Some children need the stability of a nipple in the mouth to control and propel a liquid bolus back for swallowing. If the child seems to reject the hard spout of a cup, for an easier transition, consider a soft-spout product, which is similar in texture of the nipple. If the child likes to drink from a cup while playing, this may indicate a grazing pattern that can be affecting appetite. Scheduled food/liquid intake with water between may help.)

Any siblings? Does your child eat/drink better when siblings or peers are present? Any similar feeding/GI issues in the family?

_____

_____

_____

_____

_____

(If feeding behaviors improve or worsen in the presence of others, this may indicate a behavioral component to the feeding problem. A history of GI disorders in the family should be reported to the child's physician as this may indicate a problem in the GI tract.)

Evaluation and Treatment of Pediatric Feeding Disorders: From NICU to Childhood

Page 5 • Fraker-Walbert Feeding History and Referral Guide

VIII. Referral Guide

*Any problems with reflux or vomiting? Is there any pattern to the vomiting? Is it forceful? Is it also through the nose? What comes up, is it food or bile?*_____

_____

_____

_____

(Gastroesophageal reflux does not follow a pattern, it is random and occurs whenever the lower esophageal sphincter opens and closes. It may be two hours after a meal or 20 minutes after a meal. Forceful patterned vomiting that seems to follow a cycle of occurrence, hours to weeks, or occur about the same length of time after eating is a red flag. Also note what is in the vomit and the amount that comes up when the child is vomiting.)

*Any problems with constipation or diarrhea? Any blood in the stool?*_____

_____

_____

_____

(Child should be referred to physician or pediatric gastroenterologist. Constipation can also result from low fluid intake. Some infants present with blood in the stool due to allergic colitis, however, this blood in the stool should be reported to the physician immediately.)

*Has your child had frequent colds, ear infections or upper respiratory infections?*_____

_____

_____

(Swallow evaluation may be indicated. Note: Repeating some of the medical history questions can reveal additional information about the child.)

Have you noticed any of the following when your child is eating or drinking?

- ❏ Food refusals*
- ❏ Tight, closed mouth*
- ❏ Gagging*
- ❏ Poor appetite
- ❏ Wide or watery eyes*
- ❏ Liquid/food spilling out of mouth*
- ❏ Gulpy swallows*
- ❏ Coughing*

- ❏ Choking*
- ❏ Color change with meals (pale, gray)*
- ❏ Arching*
- ❏ Crying/screaming, avoiding meal
- ❏ Long feedings*
- ❏ Fatigue with meals
   *Indicative of possible swallow dysfunction

Does your child sleep well? Wake frequently, gag or cough at night, snore or do you note mouth breathing patterns?

_____

_____

_____

(Waking at night can be indicative of hunger due to inadequate daily intake or grazing patterns, gagging or coughing may also indicate gastroesophageal reflux, snoring and mouth breathing may be signs of enlarged adenoids or nasal obstruction that could impact effective feeding.)

_____   _____

Signature   *Date*

166

Additional Resources

Inpatient Oral-Motor/Feeding Evaluation:
The Premature Infant

Name_____DOB_____DOS_____

Parent's Names_____#Siblings_____

Other Caregivers_____

Referring Physician_____

Diagnosis_____

Pre-Feeding Observations

Respiration
- ❒ Clear
- ❒ Stridor
- ❒ Labored Breathing
- ❒ Poor secretion management
- ❒ Supplemental Oxygen
- ❒ Tracheotomy: Size_____Type_____

State
- ❒ Alert
- ❒ Calm
- ❒ Drowsy
- ❒ Sleep
- ❒ Irritable
- ❒ Crying
- ❒ Inconsolable

*Pain*_____

Structural Observations and Oral Reflexes

Describe:
Lips _____
Teeth _____
Velum _____
Palate _____
Cheeks _____
Mandible _____
Tone _____

Oral Reflexes, Describe:
Root _____
Suck _____
Swallow _____
Phasic Bite _____
Transverse Tongue _____
Gag _____
Cough _____

Comments: _____
_____
_____
_____
_____

Evaluation and Treatment of Pediatric Feeding Disorders: From NICU to Childhood

Page 2 • Inpatient Oral-Motor/Feeding Evaluation: The Premature Infant

---

Non-Nutritive Suck

❑ With gloved finger: _____

_____

_____

❑ With pacifier: _____

_____

_____

Feeding Assessment

Suck/Swallow/Breathe Sequence
- ❑ Incoordinated, does not initiate sucking
- ❑ Sucking without adequate pauses for breathing
- ❑ Brief periods of coordinated sucking
- ❑ Inappropriate tongue position during feeding
- ❑ Weak, ineffective sucking, poor bolus control

- ❑ Oral spillage:
  - ___minimal_____
  - ___moderate_____
- ❑ Initially feeding well, then fatigues
- ❑ Pauses and sucking bursts of equal duration
- ❑ Coordinated suck/swallow/breathe

Feeding Red Flags
- ❑ Arching back, neck or head
- ❑ Noisy breathing patterns
- ❑ Desaturation

- ❑ ___Coughing, ___Choking, ___Gagging
- ❑ Spitting
- ❑ Vomiting

*Nutritive Sucking Describe:*_____

_____

_____

_____

_____

Nipple Used: _____

_____

Recommended Nipple: _____

_____

Attempted Feeding Interventions:

_____

_____

_____

_____

_____

_____

_____

Additional Resources

Page 3 • Inpatient Oral-Motor/Feeding Evaluation: The Premature Infant

Initial Treatment Plan: _____

_____

_____

_____

_____

_____

_____

Parent Education Results: _____

_____

_____

_____

_____

_____

_____

Next contact with family:
- ❏ Phone report
- ❏ Daily feeding sessions
- ❏ Care conference needed
- ❏ Outpatient appointment/home visit _____

_____

_____

Summary: _____

_____

_____

_____

_____

_____

_____

Recommendations:
- ❏ NPO
- ❏ Speech only to provide therapeutic feedings
- ❏ Nipple as tolerated, do not push intake
- ❏ Nipple if alert
- ❏ Nipple 1 x per shift
- ❏ Nipple every other feeding
- ❏ Nipple attempts at each scheduled feeding

Comments: _____

_____

_____

_____

_____

_____   _____
Signature   Date

Evaluation and Treatment of Pediatric Feeding Disorders: From NICU to Childhood

---

Feeding Team Clinic Evaluation & Recommendations
Summary

Name_____DOB_____

Parents/Caregivers Names_____

Address: _____

Phone _____

School _____ Grade _____ Teacher _____

Daycare Provider _____

Pediatrician/Physician _____

Reason for Referral _____

Primary Feeders _____

Feeding Clinic Summary _____

Date of Visit _____

Behavioral Psychology Consultation: ❐ Yes, ❐ No

Type of Admission: ❐ Diagnostic, ❐ Intensive Treatment, ❐ Behavioral

Admitting Diagnosis: _____

Orders: _____

_____

_____

_____

_____

Concerns: _____

_____

_____

_____

_____

Goals:_____

_____

_____

_____

_____

Planned Date of Admission: _____

_____

Physician's Signature

Additional Resources

Inpatient Daily Team Meeting Form

Patient: _____ **Date**: _____ **Day**: 1 2 3 4 5 6 7 8
Diet: ☐ regular, ☐ child diet, ☐ pureed/soft, ☐ puree, ☐ bottle-liquid only
Liquid Consistency: ☐ no restrictions, ☐ thickened: nectar-honey-milkshake
Special Instructions: _____
_____
_____

Admitting Physician: _____

Daily Plan:
Speech/Feeding Specialist: _____
- ☐ Feed patient all meals and two snacks a day, parent education after each feeding
- ☐ Evaluate, treat 1-2 times per day and continue parent education program
- ☐ Swallow study and determine safe diet, feed 1-2 times per day
- ☐ Monitor meals, parent and nurse primary feeders and start discharge planning

Nurse: _____
- ☐ General cares
- ☐ Feed evening snack
- ☐ Monitor parent with evening snack
- ☐ Medical/Behavioral observations

Occupational Therapist: _____
- ☐ See regarding positioning for feeding
- ☐ Treat for state management/sensory based feeding issues
- ☐ See regarding adaptive feeding equipment

Dietitian: _____
- ☐ Manage feeding protocols
- ☐ Calorie Counts
- ☐ Daily weights
- ☐ Parent Education
- ☐ Provide recommendations regarding appropriate foods

Social Work: _____
- ☐ Standard social history and assess area of need/appropriate referrals
- ☐ Explore financial stressors
- ☐ Family relationship evaluation
- ☐ Primary caregivers/child interaction and counseling recommendations
- ☐ Discharge Planning

Child Life Specialist: _____
- ☐ Provide activities/play time rewards after successful meals and snacks
- ☐ Educate family regarding appropriate interaction/play and toys
- ☐ Assist team with schedule
- ☐ Determine child's appropriate motivators/rewards

All team members agree with the daily treatment plan.

Team Leader_____Date_____

171

Evaluation and Treatment of Pediatric Feeding Disorders: From NICU to Childhood

Patient Name_____**Date**_____

Inpatient Daily Feeding Evaluation Form

Breakfast

Feeder: ☐ ST, ☐ OT, ☐ Nurse, ☐ Parent, ☐ Dietitian, ☐ Child Life
   ☐ Other:_____

Behaviors: ___Gagging, ___Choking, ___Coughing, ___Watery Eyes, ___Gurgly Vocal Quality, ___Color Change, ___Oral Spillage, ___Food Refusals, ___Dropping or Throwing Food, ___Pushing Food Away, ___Vomiting /Rumination, ___Crying, ___Screaming, ___Anxiety, ___Anger

Comments: _____
_____
_____
_____

AM Snack

Feeder: ☐ ST, ☐ OT, ☐ Nurse, ☐ Parent, ☐ Dietitian, ☐ Child Life
   ☐ Other:_____

Behaviors: ___Gagging, ___Choking, ___Coughing, ___Watery Eyes, ___ Gurgly Vocal Quality, ___Color Change, ___Oral Spillage, ___Poor Chewing, ___Food Refusals, ___Dropping/Throwing Food, ___Pushing Food Away, ___Vomiting / Rumination, ___Crying, ___Screaming, ___Anxiety, ___Anger

Comments: _____
_____
_____
_____

Lunch

Feeder: ☐ ST, ☐ OT, ☐ Nurse, ☐ Parent, ☐ Dietitian, ☐ Child Life
   ☐ Other:_____

Behaviors: ___Gagging, ___Choking, ___Coughing, ___Watery Eyes, ___Gurgly Vocal Quality, ___Color Change, ___Oral Spillage, ___Poor Chewing, ___Food Refusals, ___Dropping/Throwing Food, ___Pushing Food Away, Vomiting / Rumination, ___Crying, ___Screaming, ___Anxiety, ___Anger

Comments: _____
_____
_____
_____

PM Snack

Feeder: ☐ ST, ☐ OT, ☐ Nurse, ☐ Parent, ☐ Dietitian, ☐ Child Life
   ☐ Other:_____

Behaviors: ___Gagging, ___Choking, ___Coughing, ___Watery Eyes, ___Gurgly Vocal Quality, ___Color Change, ___Oral Spillage, ___Poor Chewing, ___Food Refusals, ___Dropping/Throwing Food, ___Delays, ___Pushing Food Away, Vomiting / Rumination, ___Crying, ___Screaming, ___Anxiety, ___Anger

Comments: _____
_____
_____
_____

Additional Resources

Page 2 • Inpatient Daily Feeding Evaluation Form

Dinner

Feeder: ❑ ST, ❑ OT, ❑ Nurse, ❑ Parent, ❑ Dietitian, ❑ Child Life
  ❑ Other:_____

Behaviors: ___Gagging, ___Choking, ___Watery Eyes, ___Gurgly Vocal Quality,
  ___Color Change, ___Oral Spillage, ___Poor Chewing, ___Food Refusals,
  ___Dropping/Throwing Food, ___Delays, ___Pushing Food Away, Vomiting /
  Rumination, ___Crying, ___Screaming, ___Anxiety, ___Anger

Comments: _____
_____
_____
_____

PM Snack

Feeder: ❑ ST, ❑ OT, ❑ Nurse, ❑ Parent, ❑ Dietitian, ❑ Child Life
  ❑ Other:_____

Behaviors: ___Gagging, ___Choking, ___Coughing, ___Watery Eyes, ___Gurgly
  Vocal Quality, ___Color Change, ___Oral Spillage, ___Poor Chewing, ___Food
  Refusals, ___Dropping/Throwing Food, ___Pushing Food Away, Vomiting /
  Rumination, ___Crying, ___Screaming, ___Anxiety, ___Anger

Comments: _____
_____
_____
_____

Daily Status:
- ❑ Achieved daily goals
- ❑ Did not achieve goals, additional team meeting required
- ❑ Gained weight
- ❑ Weight loss or no gain, additional team meeting required
- ❑ Parent education session
- ❑ Parent not present for education, additional team meeting required

Comments/Recommendations_____
_____
_____
_____
_____
_____
_____
_____
_____

Team Leader _____ *Date* _____

References

1. Alexander R, Oral-Motor Treatment for Infants and Young Children with Cerebral Palsy. *Seminars in Speech and Language* 1987, 8 (1), 87-100.
2. Alexander R, Boehme R and Cupps B. *Normal Development of Functional Motor Skills: The First Year of Life.* Tuscon, AZ: Therapy Skill Builders, 1993.
3. Als H, and Gilkerson L. 1995. Developmentally supportive care in the neonatal intensive care unit. *Zero to Three* 15(6): 2-10.
4. Arvedson, J and Brodsky, L. Pediatric Swallowing and Feeding: Assessment and Management. Singular Publishing Group, Inc. 1993.
5. Babbitt RL, et al: Behavioral assessment and treatment of pediatric feeding disorders. J Dev Behav Peditr 15:278-291, 1994.
6. Beauchamp GK, Cowart BJ, Moran M. Developmental changes in salt acceptability in human infants. Dev Psychobiol 1986;19:17-25.
7. Bernstein IL. Learned taste aversions in children receiving chemotherapy. Science 1978;200:1302-3.
8. Blackburn ST, and VandenBerg KA. 1998. Assessment and Management of neonatal neurobehavioral development. In *Comprehensive Neonatal Nursing: A Physiologic Perspective*, 2nds ed., Kenner C, Lott JW, and Flandermeyer AA, eds. Philadelphia: WB Saunders, 939-968.
9. Cherney L: Clinical Management of Dysphagia in Adults and Children. Aspen Publication, Inc. 1994.
10. Craig CM, et al: Modulations in breathing patterns during intermittent feeding in term infants and preterm infants with bronchopulmonary dysplasia. Dev Med Child Neurol 41:616-624, 1999.
11. Derkay CS, Schechter GL: Anatomy and Physiology of pediatric swallowing disorders. Otolaryngol Clin North Am 31:397-404, 1998.
12. Dodds WJ: Physiology of swallowing. Dysphagia 3:171-178, 1989.
13. Evans-Morris, Suzanne: Prefeeding Skills. Therapy Skill Builders, Inc.
14. Gagan RJ, Cupoli JM, Watkins AH: The families of children who fail to thrive: Preliminary investigations of parental deprivation among organic and non-organic cases. Child Abuse Negl 8:93-103, 1984.
15. Glass RP and Wolf LS. 1994. A global perspective on feeding assessment in the NICU. *American Journal of Occupational Therapy* 48(6):514-526.
16. Grunwald PC, and Becker PT. 1991. Developmental Enhancement: Implementing a program for the NICU. Neonatal Network 9 (6):29-45.
17. Hamdy S, et al: Organization and reorganization of human swallowing motor cortex: Implications for recovery after stroke. Clin Sci 99:151-157, 2000.
18. Hanlon MB, et al: Deglutition apnoea as indicator of maturation of suckle feeding in bottle-fed preterm infants. Dev Med Child Neurol 39:534-542, 1997.
19. Kedesky, Jurgen and Budd, Karen. 1998. *Childhood Feeding Disorders Biobehavioral Assessment and Intervention.* Paul H. Brookes Publishing Co.
20. Kunz J and Finkel A: The American Medical Association Medical Guide. Random House 1987.
21. Gaining and Growing: Assuring Nutritional Care of Preterm Infants.

22. Illingworth RS, Lister JL: The critical or sensitive period, with special reference to certain feeding problems in infants and children. J Pediatr 65:839-848, 1964.
23. Lawrence R: The Clinician's role in teaching proper infant feeding techniques. J Pediatr 1995;126:S112-7.
24. Logemann J: Evaluation and Treatment of Swallowing Disorders. Pro-Ed, Inc. 1998
25. Leonard, S., Bower, C, Petterson B, Leonard, H, Medical Aspects of School-aged Children with Down Syndrome. Dev Med Child Neurol 1999 Oct; 41 (10): 683-8
26. Link DT, et al: Pediatric laryngopharyngeal sensory testing during flexible endoscopic evaluation of swallowing: Feasible and correlative. Ann Otol Rhinol Laryngol 109(10 Pt1):899-905, 2000.
27. Lucas B, Nardella M, Feucht S: Cost considerations: The benefits of nutrition services for a case series of children with special health care needs in Washington State. Dev Iss 17:1-4, 1999.
28. Mathew OP, Belan M, Thoppil CK: Sucking patterns of neonates during bottle feeding: Comparison of different nipple units. Am J Perinatol 9:265-269, 1992.
29. McCain GC. 1997. Behavioral state activity during nipple feeding for preterm infants. Neonatal *Network* 16(5):43-47. *Journal of Obstetric, Gynecologic and Neonatal Nursing* 22(2): 147-155.
30. Meier PP. Breastfeeding Your Premature Infant. 1997a. Columbus, OH: Ross Laboratories.
31. Meier PP. Suck-breathe Patterning During Bottle and Breastfeeding for Preterm Infants. Major Controversies in Infant Nutrition (pp. 9-20), TJ David, Ed: International Congress and Symposium Series 215. *London: Royal Society of Medicine Press*, 1996.
32. Meier PP and Brown LP. Strategies to Assist Breastfeeding in Preterm Infants. *Recent Advances in Pediatrics*, 15, TJ David, Ed. 1997b, pp. 137-150. London: Churchill-Livingstone Press.
33. Meier P, Engstrom J, Mangurten H, et al. Breastfeeding Support Services in the Neonatal Intensive Care Unit. JOGNN 22:338, 1993.
34. Meier, P, Vasan U, Meier W, et al. Lactoengineering of Own Mothers' Milk for Preterm Infant Feeding. (Manuscript in preparation). 1997.
35. Mbonda E, Claus D, Bonnier C, Evrard, P, Gadisseux J, Lyon G: Prolonged dysphasia caused by congenital pharyngeal dysfunction. J Pediatr 1995;126:923-7.
36. Neifert, M, Lawrence, R, Seacat J: Nipple confusion: toward a formal definition. J Pediatr 1995; 126:S125-9.
37. Newman L, Keckley C, Peterson M, Hamner A: Swallowing Function and Medical Diagnoses in Infants Suspected of Dysphasia. Pediatrics 2001;108(6).
38. Nursing Mothers' Association of Australia ISBN Revised 1997. Breastfeeding Your Child with Down Syndrome.
39. Pridham KF, et al. 1993. Nipple feeding for preterm infants with bronchopulmonary dysplasia. Enhancement: Implementing a program for the NICU.
40. Rudolph C, Link DT: Feeding Disorders in Infants and Children. Pediatr Clin North Am Volume 49:Number 1, Feb 2002.

41. Rudolph CD, et all: Guidelines for evaluation and treatment of gastroesophageal reflux in infants and children. J Pediatr Gastroenterol Nutr 32(suppl 2):1-31, 2001.
42. Schwarz S, Corredor J, Fisher-Medina J, Cohen J, Rabinowitz S: Diagnosis and Treatment of Feeding Disorders in Children with Developmental Disabilities. Amer Acad Pediatr Vol 108, Number 3, Sept 2001.
43. Sibai BM, Ramadan MK, Chari RS, Friedman SA. Pregnancies complicated by HELLP Syndrome: Subsequent pregnancy outcome and long-term prognosis. *American Journal of Obstetrics and Gynecology* 172: 125-9, 1995.
44. Shahid S, Allen E, Shell R, Hruschak J, Iram D, Castile R, McCoy K: Chronic Aspiration without gastroesophageal reflux as a cause of chronic respiratory symptoms in neurologically normal infants. American College of Chest Physicians Vol 120, number 4, October 2001.
45. Shaker CS. 1990. Nipple feeding premature infants: A different perspective. *Neonatal Network* 8(5):9-17.
46. Shivpuri CR, et al. 1983. Decreased ventilation in preterm infants during oral feeding. *Journal of Pediatrics* 103 (2):285-289.
47. Sullivan PB, Reilly S, Skuse D: Characteristics and management of feeding problems of young children with cerebral palsy. Dev Med Child Neurol 34:379-388, 1996.
48. Trachtenbarg, M.D., and Golemon, M.D. Care of the Premature Infant: Monitoring Growth and Development Copyright 1999 American Academy of Pediatrics.
49. Tully S, Yehuda B, Bradley R: Abnormal tympanography after supine bottle feeding. J Pediatr 1995;126:S105-11.
50. Vandenberg KA. 1990. Nippling management of the sick neonate in the ICU: The disorganized feeder. *Neonatal Network* 9 (1): 9-16.
51. Vazques JL: Feeding difficulties in the first days of life: findings on upper gastrointestinal series and the role of the videofluoroscopic swallowing study. Pediatr Radiol- 01-Dec-1999; 29(12): 894-6.
52. Vitellas K, Bennett W, Bova J, et al: Radiographic manifestations of eosinophilic gastroenteritis. Abdom Imaging20:406-43, 1995.
53. Vogel S. Oral motor and feeding problems in tube fed infant: suggested treatment strategies for occupational therapists. In: Cromwell FS, ed. Occupational therapy for people with eating dysfunctions. New York: Haworth Press, 1986:63-79.
54. Wolf LS and Glass RP. 1992. *Feeding and Swallowing Disorders in Infancy.* Tucson: Therapy Skill Builders.